A H lockwood
10. HAMMELTON Road
BROMLEY

Sylvester method.
stretcher drill

Sussex

FIRST AID TO THE INJURED

THE AUTHORISED TEXTBOOK
OF THE

ST. JOHN AMBULANCE ASSOCIATION

BEING THE AMBULANCE DEPARTMENT OF

The Grand Priory in the British Realm of the
Venerable Order of the Hospital of St. John of Jerusalem

THIRTY-NINTH EDITION. FIRST IMPRESSION (100,000) 1937

Price 2/- net; by Post, 2/2d.

PUBLISHED BY
THE ST. JOHN AMBULANCE ASSOCIATION,
ST. JOHN'S GATE, CLERKENWELL, LONDON, E.C. 1.

CLERKENWELL 664

L.M.R.—12/37.   COPYRIGHT.

PREVIOUS PUBLICATIONS.

CONTENTS.

APPENDICES.

REFERENCE No. 58
1937

SYLLABUS OF INSTRUCTION—ADULT COURSE.

· A course of instruction shall extend over a minimum of twelve hours, and only members of the medical profession are recognised as Instructors. The Surgeon Instructor usually prefers to divide the course of instruction into six weekly lectures, each of two hours' duration, devoting the first hour to theory and the second to practical instruction in the application of dressings, bandages and splints, compression of arteries, artificial respiration, hand-seats and lifting and carrying injured persons on stretchers. If preferred, the Surgeon Instructor may divide the course into twelve lectures each of one hour's duration, or as convenient.

FIRST LECTURE.

Outline of First Aid.

Principles of First Aid.

Structure and Functions of the Body. *

Shock.

Dressings and Bandages.

Practical Instruction.—Dressings, and the application of the Triangular Bandage to the Head, Chest, Back, Shoulder, Elbow, Hand, Hip, Knee and Foot. Arm Slings (Large, Small and St. John).

*NOTE.—When possible a skeleton should be used. Too much time should not, however, be spent on instruction in anatomical and physiological details. Lecturers and Examiners are particularly requested to remember that it is " First Aid " that has to be taught and tested, and not anatomy and physiology.

SECOND LECTURE.

Fractures.—Causes, varieties, signs, symptoms, and general rules for treatment. Special Fractures.

Injuries to Joints and Muscles.—Dislocations, Sprains and Strains.

Practical Instruction.—Treatment of Fractures.

THIRD LECTURE.

Circulation of the Blood.—General description of the Heart, Blood Vessels and Circulation of the Blood.

Wounds and Hæmorrhage.—Wounds accompanied by Arterial Hæmorrhage. Situation of the main Arteries—pressure points. Wounds accompanied by Capillary or Venous Hæmorrhage. Varicose Veins. Snake Bite and Hydrophobia.

Hæmorrhage from Internal Organs.—Hæmorrhage from special regions—the Mouth, Nose and Ear. Bruises.

Practical Instruction.—Compression of Arteries.

FOURTH LECTURE.

The Respiratory System.—Brief description of the Respiratory organs—natural breathing. Artificial Respiration by Schafer's and Silvester's methods.

The Nervous System.—Brief description of Motor, Sensory and Sympathetic Systems.

Insensibility.—When breathing is absent (Asphyxia); when breathing is present and there are Convulsions; when breathing is present and there are no Convulsions.

Practical Instruction.—Artificial Respiration.

FIFTH LECTURE.

Poisons.—General classification and treatment. Poisons which require special treatment.

Miscellaneous Injuries.—Scalds and Burns. Stings. Frost Bite. Rupture. Foreign bodies in Eye, Ear, Nose or Stomach.

Practical Instruction.—Treatment of Fractures and Hæmorrhage.

SIXTH LECTURE.

Routine Examination of a Patient.

Preparation for the Reception of Accident Cases.

Transport of Injured Persons.—Hand-seats and, for males only, Stretcher.

Practical Instruction.—Hand-seats and, for males only, Stretcher Exercises.

LIST OF ILLUSTRATIONS.

8

A*

APPENDICES.

INTRODUCTION.

The St. John Ambulance Association is a Foundation of the Grand Priory of the Venerable Order of St. John, and came into existence in 1877, although as early as 1872 tentative efforts to introduce an ambulance service in the Potteries had been made.

Certificates of proficiency in First Aid after attendance at lectures and examination were granted in 1877 and the first manual of instruction was published in 1878, having been written for the Association by the late Surgeon-Major Peter Shepherd, M.B. So keenly was the work taken up, especially by miners, policemen and railwaymen, that in 1879 the Association introduced a system of re-examination for further awards. The experience of a few years soon showed that there could be no finality in the scheme of the Association. Those who had received certificates and medallions exhibited a keen desire to utilise their knowledge in the service of the public. Many of them accordingly banded themselves together in units at various centres, and provided ambulance stations at National and International Exhibitions and other places where large crowds assembled. Thus originated the St. John Ambulance Brigade, which was eventually established by the Order of St. John in 1887.

In the meanwhile the Association had turned its attention to the manufacture and improvement of ambulance litters and stretchers. These latter were so designed as to fit all methods of transport and even in those early days it was possible for a patient to be conveyed across Europe without needing removal from the stretcher, or suffering from variations in transport.

No greater tribute to the work of the Association could have been paid than the granting of the Charter to the Order of St. John in 1888 by Her Majesty Queen Victoria.

Since its inception over sixty years ago the Association has issued to successful students in all parts of the world over two million certificates, which are recognised by the Home Office, Board of Trade, Admiralty, War Office and other Government Departments and Civil Authorities.

The St. John Ambulance Brigade, now numbering at home and overseas more than 100,000 members, is universally recognised as a necessary unit of civil life, ready to serve on all occasions where accidents are liable to occur. The Brigade also provides fully trained persons for the Royal Naval Auxiliary Sick Berth Reserve, the Military Hospitals Reserve and Voluntary Aid Detachments.

PREFACE.

At the request of the Ambulance Committee of the Order of St. John, we have revised the First Aid Textbook of the St. John Ambulance Association. Our task has not been easy, for since the last revision in 1928 three questions have been the subject of much difference of opinion, namely, the scope of First Aid, the treatment of burns, and the method of transporting a patient with a spinal injury.

As regards the first, owing to the tendency in some quarters to encourage the First-Aider to encroach on the duties of a trained nurse, and even of a doctor, we have thought it necessary to introduce a stricter definition of First Aid.

On the subject of burns we are unanimously agreed that the treatment of extensive burns and scalds by tannic acid is a matter of skilled technique, and is beyond the scope of First Aid.

With regard to spinal injuries, we have consulted various authorities, and, although we have not found unanimity among them, we have, nevertheless, decided to modify the methods to be observed by First-Aiders in the transport of such cases.

Chapters on Shock and its treatment and on the Routine Examination of a Patient and many new illustrations have been added.

We are greatly indebted to Dr. Hamilton Fairley for writing the sections on snake bite and hydrophobia; and to many correspondents for their helpful criticisms and suggestions.

We have discussed with the Royal Life Saving Society the subject of artificial respiration, and are in agreement with that Society that no method is so effective as Schafer's, and we are indebted to the Society for their help and for permission to reproduce illustrations very closely resembling those which appear in the Society's Manual.

A. N. CAHUSAC (Chairman).
W. E. AUDLAND, M.R.C.S.
R. B. DUNCAN, M.D.
A. C. W. KNOX, M.B.
A. T. LAKIN, M.B.
I. G. MODLIN, M.D.

September, 1937.

Chapter I.

OUTLINE OF FIRST AID.

What First Aid is.

The science of First Aid to the Injured is based on fundamental principles of practical medicine and surgery, a knowledge of which, in cases of accident and sudden illness, enables trained persons to render such skilled assistance as will preserve life, promote recovery or prevent aggravation of the injury or condition until the arrival of the doctor or during transport.

First Aid is definitely limited to the assistance rendered at the time of the emergency with such material as may be available. It is not intended that the First-Aider should take the place of the doctor, and it must be clearly understood that the re-dressing of injuries and other after-treatment is outside the scope of First Aid.

The First-Aider's responsibilities end as soon as medical aid is available; but he should stand by after making his report to the doctor in case he can be of further assistance.

NECESSARY QUALIFICATIONS OF A FIRST-AIDER.

In order to render the skilled assistance required the First-Aider should be—

(a) **Observant,** that he may note the causes and signs of injury.

(b) **Tactful,** that he may, without thoughtless questions, learn the symptoms and history of the case, and secure the confidence of the patient and bystanders.

(c) **Resourceful,** that he may use to the best advantage whatever is at hand to prevent further damage and assist Nature's efforts to repair the mischief already done.

(d) **Dextrous,** that he may handle a patient without causing unnecessary pain, and use appliances efficiently and neatly.

(e) **Explicit,** that he may give clear instructions to the patient or the bystanders how best to assist him.

(f) **Discriminating,** that he may decide which of several injuries should be treated first.

(g) **Persevering,** that he may continue his efforts, though not at first successful.

(h) **Sympathetic,** that he may give real comfort and encouragement to the suffering.

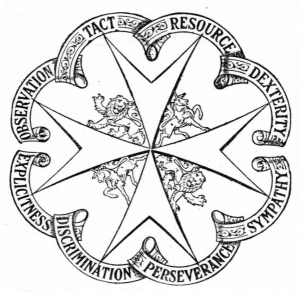

FIG. 1.—THE EIGHT-POINTED AMBULANCE CROSS.

ESSENTIALS OF FIRST AID.

In First Aid to the Injured it is essential :—

(a) To determine the nature of the case
requiring attention so far as is necessary
for intelligent and efficient treatment,—in
other words, to make a sufficient diagnosis
for the purposes falling within the province
of the First-Aider.

(b) To decide on the character and extent of
the treatment to be given.

(c) To apply the treatment most suited to
the circumstances until medical aid is
available.

Everything that has any bearing on the case
should be considered :—

1. The Patient or Patients.—The position
assumed by the patient, either voluntarily or by
force of circumstances, should not escape observation. More than one patient may need assistance,
and discrimination will be necessary to ensure that
the most pressing needs of each receive prompt
attention.

2. Signs, Symptoms and History.—By
" signs " are meant any differences from the normal
condition of the patient, such as pallor, congestion,
swelling, deformity, which can be noted by the
direct use of the senses, sight, touch, smell and

hearing. "Symptoms" are the sensations of the patient such as pain, numbness, giddiness, hunger, which he can, if conscious, describe; while "history," which may be obtained from the patient or from witnesses, means the circumstances attending the accident or sudden illness, such as a collision or fall or being subject to a particular disease. Symptoms are less reliable than signs, as one patient will make light of a very severe injury while another will make the most of a trifle ; and history must be considered trustworthy in proportion to the reliability of the source whence it is obtained.

Symptoms taken alone are not of much value for diagnosis, but they have their uses, as warnings of something wrong, as guides to the seat of mischief, or, in many cases, by their abatement or increased severity, as indications whether the treatment given is effective.

Symptoms when considered in conjunction with the history of the case are distinctly more valuable for purposes of diagnosis.

When to the above there is added information gained by the observation of definite signs, the diagnosis rests upon a solid basis.

3. The Cause or Causes.— When a cause is known, a conclusion, more or less accurate, may be

drawn as to its probable effects. But it must be remembered :—

(a) That a cause may have more than one effect. For example, two or more injuries may result from one accident.

(b) That the effect or effects may be direct or indirect. For example, a blood-vessel may break in the head, causing insensibility (direct effect). The patient will fall as the result of the bursting of the blood-vessel and a further injury may occur as the result of the fall (indirect effect).

(c) That the cause may be still active. For example, a foreign body in the throat may continue to impede breathing as long as it remains there.

4. Surroundings.—These will exercise a most important bearing on the treatment to be given, and therefore require careful consideration on the following lines :—

(a) **Possible sources of danger,** such as fire, moving machinery, electric wires, poisonous gases, a restive horse, slippery objects, may be present and necessitate the protection not only of the patient but also of the First-Aider and of others.

(b) **Possible clues to diagnosis**, such as a broken ladder, stains of blood, escaping gas, bottles, etc., may afford useful suggestions. Objects suspected of having some connection with the patient's injury or illness should, compatibly with the pressing needs of the emergency, be examined and preserved for future reference.

(c) **Help available** depends in the first place on the presence or nearness of persons capable of helping, and in the second place upon the discrimination, explicitness and tact with which their efforts are directed. By the exercise of these qualities an inquisitive crowd may be so controlled and instructed as to be of vital assistance to the patient.

(d) **Appliances available.**—Appliances may be at hand, but if not, the First-Aider must be resourceful in utilizing such means of improvising as may be available. The directions and illustrations which are given throughout this book are intended as a standard of treatment. It will frequently be impossible, for lack of appliances, to carry out the treatment exactly in the manner indicated. In such cases it will be necessary to comply with the principles of treatment in the best manner consistent with the actual circumstances.

(*e*) **Shelter.**—This word must be understood as including an extra wrap, or an umbrella, etc., as a temporary protection against the inclemency of the weather or fierce rays of the sun, as well as a shed, a private house, or a hospital.

(*f*) **Means of transport available.**—Consideration of the best means of transport to shelter involves questions of appliances, length of journey, the nature of the ground to be traversed, and the best disposal of the help available for removing the patient. If the patient is to be taken to his home a tactful message thereto might enable suitable accommodation to be made, and in any case would be an act of kindness to those concerned.

———————

Chapter II.

PRINCIPLES OF FIRST AID.

The following Principles are the basis of all First Aid treatment. It is therefore of the greatest importance that the First-Aider should understand them thoroughly and apply them effectively:—

1. Death is not to be assumed because signs of life are absent.—It may happen that even a doctor is unable to say positively whether a patient is alive or dead; far less can the First-Aider form a decision. It is much better to treat a dead body than to allow a living person to die for want of First Aid.

2. Remove the cause of injury or danger whenever possible, or, when more expedient, remove the patient from the cause.

3. Severe hæmorrhage must receive immediate attention, no matter what other injuries are present.

4. Air.—The patient must be in a position in which breathing is possible; the air passages must be free from obstruction. If breathing has ceased immediate measures must be taken to restore it.

5. Warmth.—Keep the patient warm, and so arrest the fall of temperature and lessen shock. This may be done by wrapping the patient in blankets, coats or rugs, and by applying hot water bottles or hot bricks to the body. Hot water bottles and bricks must be covered with flannel and the heat tested on the bare forearm.

6. Rest.—A restful position of the body will assist the vital functions. The position assumed by the patient should not be thoughtlessly altered. Support of the injured part will help to prevent further damage. The use of pillows in this connection is much to be commended.

7. When the skin is broken the wound should be immediately covered with a clean dressing.

8. When a bone is broken no attempt must be made to move the patient until the bone has been rendered as immovable as practicable, unless life is in danger from some other cause.

9. Poisons swallowed should be got rid of, or, when that is inexpedient, neutralised.

10. The best means of transport must be arranged, and provision made for proper care when the patient is brought to shelter.

11. Removal of Clothing.—Uncover the patient as little as possible since exposure increases shock ; but if it is needful to remove clothing, it should not be cut unnecessarily. The following rules will be of service :—

> Coat : Slip the coat off the shoulders, then remove from the sound side first, and if necessary, slit up the seam of the sleeve on the injured side.
>
> Shirt and Vest : Slit down the front and remove as the coat.
>
> Trousers : Slit up the outer seam.
>
> Boot : Steady the ankle and undo the laces.
>
> Sock : Cut off.

12. Stimulants.—When the patient is able to swallow, strong tea or coffee with plenty of sugar, meat extracts or milk, as hot as can be drunk, or a teaspoonful of sal volatile in half a tumbler of water may be given. Ampoules of ammonia may be crushed in a handkerchief and the vapour inhaled. Smelling salts, the strength of which should first be tested, may be held to the nose. Sprinkling the face with cold and hot water alternately, warmth applied to the pit of the stomach and over the heart, and vigorous friction of the limbs upwards have a stimulating effect. It is incorrect to suppose that alcohol is the only form of stimulant.

Too frequent use of spirits is made to restore a patient after an accident, often with serious results ; **the administration of alcohol must therefore be withheld until ordered by the doctor.**

13. The First-Aider must on no account take upon himself the duties and responsibilities of a doctor.—At times an apparently slight injury is accompanied by grave danger or may easily be aggravated by rough or unskilful treatment, which may actually cause loss of life.

The importance of making early provision for medical aid cannot be too strongly insisted on. Discrimination must be exercised as to advising the patient to see a doctor, sending for the doctor or taking the patient to him or to hospital. When sending for a doctor, state the nature of the case, the whereabouts of the patient, and, if it is intended to move him at once, the destination and the route to be followed. Written particulars are safer than a verbal message.

PROVISION FOR **MEDICAL AID** AND THE **TREATMENT OF SHOCK** ARE ESSENTIAL PARTS OF FIRST AID. AS THESE TWO MAXIMS MUST BE FOLLOWED **IN ALL CASES,** IT WILL BE UNNECESSARY TO REFER TO THEM AGAIN EXCEPT TO EMPHASISE THEIR URGENCY.

CHAPTER III.

STRUCTURE AND FUNCTIONS OF THE BODY.

In order to understand fully the principles of First Aid it is necessary that something should be known of the structure of the body (anatomy), and the functions of some of the more important organs and systems (physiology).

THE STRUCTURE OF THE BODY.

THE SKELETON.

The human body is moulded upon a bony framework (the skeleton) which serves :—

    1.—To give shape and firmness to the body.

    2.—To afford attachment to the muscles.

    3.—To protect important organs, as in the skull, chest and abdomen.

THE SKULL.

The Bones of the Skull are arranged in two groups, those of the brain case (Cranium) and those of the face.

The Boundaries of the Cranium are the vault or dome, the rounded portion forming the top of the head; the front or brow; the back of the head, where the greatest extent of brain is situated, and where therefore the cranium is widest and deepest; the sides or temples. The base of the skull is hidden from view by the bones of the face and of the spinal column; in it are numerous openings for the passage of blood vessels and nerves; through the largest opening the brain and spinal cord are continuous.

The Bones of the Head and Face, with the exception of the lower jaw, are firmly united, so that movement between them is impossible. The cavities of the nose and of the eye sockets (Orbits) are formed by the bones of the cranium and of the face conjointly. The mouth cavity is formed between the upper and lower jaws, the palate being the bony roof of the mouth which separates it from the nasal cavity above.

The Lower Jaw consists of :—

(a) A horizontal portion in which are the sockets for the teeth.

(b) Vertical portions terminating on either side at the joint between the lower jaw and the base of the skull situated immediately in front of the ear.

The angle of the jaw indicates the junction of the horizontal and vertical portions.

THE BACK-BONE OR SPINE (VERTEBRAL COLUMN).

The Spine (Fig. 2) is composed of bones called vertebræ. Each consists of a body or bony mass in front, from the sides of which processes extend backwards and unite to form the spinal canal, which encloses the spinal cord (Figs. 3 and 4).

The Vertebræ, 33 in all, are grouped into regions in each of which they are known by numbers, counting downwards :—

1.—In the neck 7 Cervical vertebræ. The first vertebra (Atlas) forms a joint with the base of the skull, at which the nodding movement of the head takes place ; the second (Axis), by means of the joint between it and the atlas, permits the side-to-side movements of the head.

2.—In the back 12 Thoracic vertebræ, to which the ribs are attached.

3.—In the loin 5 Lumbar vertebræ.

4.—The rump-bone (Sacrum) consists of 5 Sacral vertebræ united in adults as a solid mass.

5.—The tail-bone (Coccyx) consists of 4 vertebræ joined together.

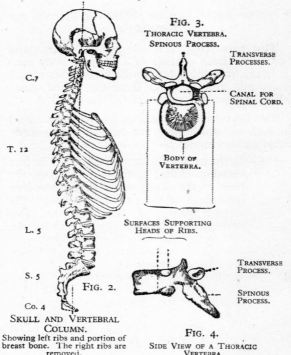

FIG. 3.
THORACIC VERTEBRA.
SPINOUS PROCESS.

TRANSVERSE PROCESSES.

CANAL FOR SPINAL CORD.

BODY OF VERTEBRA.

C. 7

T. 12

L. 5

S. 5

Co. 4

FIG. 2.

SKULL AND VERTEBRAL COLUMN.
Showing left ribs and portion of breast bone. The right ribs are removed.

SURFACES SUPPORTING HEADS OF RIBS.

TRANSVERSE PROCESS.

SPINOUS PROCESS.

FIG. 4.
SIDE VIEW OF A THORACIC VERTEBRA.

Between the bodies of the vertebræ, in the upper three regions, are interposed thick pieces of gristle (cartilage), which allow of free movement to the column as a whole, and help to break the shock of any sudden force applied to the spine (for example, when falling from a height on the feet). The whole spine is strapped together by bands of strong fibrous tissue (ligaments) reaching its entire length.

THE RIBS AND BREAST-BONE.

The Ribs consist of twelve pairs of curved bones extending from the thoracic vertebræ to the front of the body, and are known by numbers—first, second, etc., commencing from above. The ribs are not bony throughout their entire length, but at a short distance from the front the bony material ends, and cartilage takes its place. The upper seven pairs, called the " true " ribs, are attached by their cartilages to the **Breast-bone** (Sternum), a dagger-shaped bone with the point downwards, just above the pit of the stomach. The lower five pairs of ribs are called " false." Of these the upper three pairs are attached by cartilage to the ribs immediately above them. The last two pairs are unattached in front and are called " floating." The ribs enclose the chest and serve to protect the lungs, heart, liver, stomach, spleen, etc.

THE UPPER LIMBS.

The Shoulder-bones are the Collar-bone (Clavicle) and the Shoulder-blade (Scapula).

The Collar-bone can be felt on either side beneath the skin at the lower and front part of the neck as a narrow curved rod about the thickness of a finger. Its inner end is attached to the upper part of the breast-bone, and its outer end joins with the shoulder-blade.

The Shoulder-blade lies at the upper and outer part of the back of the chest, and forms joints with the collar-bone and the bone of the arm.

The Bone of the Arm (Humerus) reaches from the shoulder to the elbow.

In the **Forearm** are two bones, one on the outer, or thumb side (Radius) and the other on the inner, or little finger side (Ulna). Both bones reach from the elbow to the wrist, and they change their relative position with every turn of the hand (Figs. 5 and 6).

The Hand is composed of :—

1.—The bones of the wrist (Carpus), eight in number, arranged in two rows of four.

2.—The framework of the palm (Metacarpus); five bones which form the knuckles and support the bones of the fingers.

3.—The finger-bones (Phalanges), three in each finger, and two in the thumb.

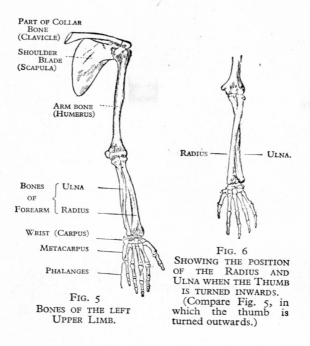

PART OF COLLAR
BONE
(CLAVICLE)

SHOULDER
BLADE
(SCAPULA)

ARM BONE
(HUMERUS)

BONES { ULNA
OF
FOREARM { RADIUS

WRIST (CARPUS)

METACARPUS

PHALANGES

RADIUS ——— ULNA.

FIG. 5
BONES OF THE LEFT
UPPER LIMB.

FIG. 6
SHOWING THE POSITION
OF THE RADIUS AND
ULNA WHEN THE THUMB
IS TURNED INWARDS.
(Compare Fig. 5, in
which the thumb is
turned outwards.)

B

THE PELVIS AND LOWER LIMBS.

The Pelvis.—The large basin-like mass of bone attached to the lower part of the spine is called the Pelvis and is composed of the two haunch-bones, the sacrum and the coccyx. The haunch-bones meet at the front (Pubes) in the middle line, only a small piece of cartilage intervening, but behind, the sacrum is placed between them. The pelvis supports the abdomen and its contents, and provides the deep sockets for the hip-joints.

The Thigh-bone (Femur) reaches from the hip to the knee-joint. Its shaft is stout, rounded, and arched forwards ; the upper end presents a rounded head, supported on a neck which projects inwards, to fit into the socket of the haunch bone ; the lower end broadens and enters into the formation of the knee-joint.

The Knee-cap (Patella) is a flat triangular bone lying with its base upwards in front of the knee-joint immediately beneath the skin.

The Bones of the Leg are the Shin-bone (Tibia) and the Brooch-bone (Fibula). The **Shin-bone** extends from the knee to the ankle, in both of which joints it plays an important part : its sharp edge can be felt immediately beneath the skin of the front of the leg. The **Brooch-bone** lies on the

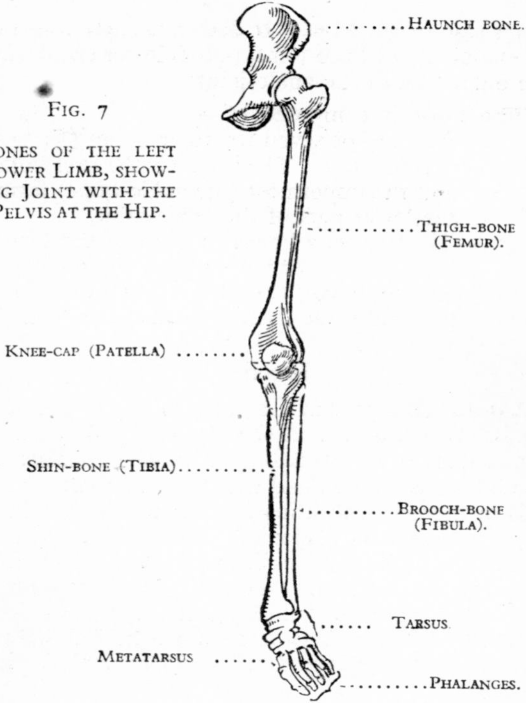

.... HAUNCH BONE.

FIG. 7

BONES OF THE LEFT
LOWER LIMB, SHOW-
ING JOINT WITH THE
PELVIS AT THE HIP.

.... THIGH-BONE
(FEMUR).

KNEE-CAP (PATELLA) ....

SHIN-BONE (TIBIA)..........

.... BROOCH-BONE
(FIBULA).

.... TARSUS.

METATARSUS ......

.... PHALANGES.

outer side of the tibia. It does not enter into the formation of the knee-joint, but its lower end forms the outer part of the ankle-joint.

The Foot is composed of —

1.—A group of seven irregular bones (Tarsus) at the instep. The largest is the heel-bone, and the uppermost (the ankle-bone) forms the lower part of the ankle-joint.

2.—The five long bones in front of the tarsus (Metatarsus) which support the toes.

3.—The toe-bones (Phalanges), two in the big toe, and three in each of the other toes.

JOINTS.

A **Joint** is formed at the junction of two or more bones. In joints such as the hip, knee, elbow, etc., the surfaces of the bones are covered by cartilage, which lessens friction and the shock of a fall. The ends of the bones forming a joint are enclosed in a bag of strong tissue (capsule). This is strengthened by bands of similar tissue (ligaments) which hold the bones in position and allow of free movement. Within the capsule is a lining (synovial membrane), its function being to secrete fluid (synovial fluid), which is always present inside the joint and acts as a lubricant.

The following examples of joints are given :—

1.—**Ball and Socket Joints** (Fig. 8), in which the rounded head of one bone fits into a cup-shaped cavity formed by the other bone entering into the joint, such as the Shoulder and Hip. In these joints very free movement is allowed and they are frequently dislocated.

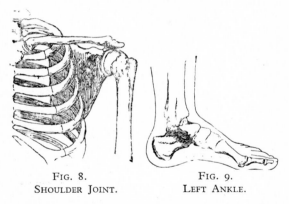

FIG. 8.
SHOULDER JOINT.

FIG. 9.
LEFT ANKLE.

2.—**Hinge Joints** (Fig. 9), in which the surfaces of the bones are moulded to each other in such a manner as to permit only bending (flexion) and straightening (extension), such as the Elbow, Knee and Ankle. In these joints considerable force is necessary to cause a dislocation.

In the knee-joint are two flat crescentic pieces of cartilage (semi-lunar cartilages) which lie on the upper end of the tibia, and deepen the surface for the rounded ends of the femur. In sudden wrenches of the knee, such as are met with in football and other games or in slipping off a step, these cartilages may be displaced or torn.

THE TISSUES.

The Muscles (red flesh) of the body are classified into two groups—voluntary and involuntary.

The Voluntary Muscles are met with in the limbs, the head and neck, and the walls of the trunk. They are attached to the bones either directly or by strong bands of white fibrous tissue (tendons), and have the power of contracting, i.e., getting shorter and thicker. They cause all the movements of the body and limbs, and are controlled by the brain, which sends messages (impulses) through the nerves to any muscle or group of muscles which it wishes to call into action. In this way all movements, such as walking or swallowing, are performed. (Cerebro-spinal system, see page 152.)

The Involuntary Muscles are met with in the walls of the stomach and intestines, in the air passages, and in most of the internal organs and blood vessels ; and, in a special form, in the heart. They are not under the influence of the will, but continue their work during the hours of sleep ; their functions are regulated by a separate set of nerves (Sympathetic System, see page 153).

Connective Tissue consists of yellow elastic and white fibrous tissue intermixed in varying proportions. It is present in many parts of the body and forms a layer between the skin and underlying flesh all over the body, fat being contained between its meshes, often in large quantities. The chief use of the connective tissue is to bind parts together.

The Skin covers the whole of the body and protects the underlying structures. It consists of two layers, the outer and hard layer (cuticle) and the inner layer (true skin or dermis). In the latter are numerous glands which secrete sweat ; this consists of water and impurities from the blood, the evaporation of which from the surface of the skin cools and helps to regulate the temperature of the body.

THE TRUNK AND ITS CONTENTS.

The Trunk is divided by a large arched muscular partition (**Diaphragm**) into two large cavities.

The upper cavity, the **Chest** (Thorax) is bounded in front by the breast-bone ; behind by the spine ;

below by the diaphragm, and is encircled by the ribs. It contains the **Heart** and **Lungs.**

The lower cavity, the **Abdomen,** is bounded above by the diaphragm; below by the pelvis; behind by the lumbar vertebræ; and in front and at the sides by muscular walls (Fig. 10). It contains several important organs, namely the **Stomach,** just below the diaphragm towards the left side; the **Liver,** in the upper part of the abdomen, where it is mostly covered by the right lower ribs; the **Spleen,** covered by the ribs at the upper part of the left side of the abdomen; the **Pancreas,** behind the stomach; the **Intestines,** which occupy the greater part of the cavity of the abdomen; the **Kidneys,** at the back, one at each side, in the region of the loin; and the **Bladder** which lies to the front in the pelvis.

FUNCTIONS OF THE BODY.

The body requires fuel and new material to repair its wear and tear. These are obtained from the food eaten—fats such as cream and butter, and starches such as bread and vegetables, to provide the fuel; and nitrogenous foods such as meat, beans and cheese, to make good the wear and tear. These are digested in the mouth, stomach and bowels, and

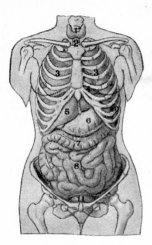 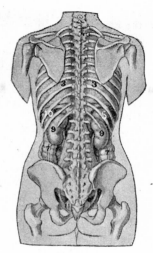

FIG. 10.   FIG. 11.

ORGANS OF THE CHEST AND ABDOMEN.
(Front view.)   (Back view.)

1.—ŒSOPHAGUS OR GULLET.   2.—TRACHEA OR WINDPIPE.   3-3.—RIGHT AND LEFT LUNGS.   4.—HEART.   5.—LIVER.   6.—STOMACH.   7.—LARGE INTESTINE.   8.—SMALL INTESTINE.   9-9.—RIGHT AND LEFT KIDNEYS.   10.—SPLEEN.   11.—BLADDER.

Reproduced by kind permission of Messrs. S. H. Camp and Company, Michigan, U.S.A.

B*

are changed so that they can be easily absorbed by the blood. Oxygen, too, is necessary to support life. This is obtained from the air we breathe in respiration, and is absorbed in the lungs. The waste products are removed through the skin, lungs, kidneys and bowels.

The great carrier is the blood, which conveys the fresh supplies of oxygen and nourishment to the whole of the body from the lungs and organs of digestion, and also the waste products to the organs of excretion.

All these movements and functions of the body are regulated and controlled by two systems of **Nerves,** the Cerebro-spinal and the Sympathetic.

CHAPTER IV.

SHOCK.

Shock is a condition of sudden depression of the nervous system resulting from, and occurring after every case of accident or sudden illness. It may vary from a slight feeling of faintness to a condition of collapse in which the vital forces of the body are so exhausted that death may result.

The injury itself is the primary cause of the condition ; and, in many cases, the shock will be overcome by rest and warmth whilst the injury is being treated. There are, however, other cases such as severe crushes, abdominal injuries, burns and the like, where shock develops rapidly and becomes the grave danger to life ; in these cases, **shock must be treated first,** but precautions must be taken to prevent any aggravation of the original injury.

Shock will be increased by :—
   (1) Loss of blood :
   (2) Exposure to cold :
   (3) Severe pain :
   (4) Mental anxiety.

The first indications of the onset of shock are pallor of the face and lips, with " beads of cold sweat " appearing on the forehead, and the skin cold and clammy : the pulse becomes rapid and feeble, and later may be imperceptible at the wrist : the breathing is shallow ; the temperature of the body falls. The patient complains of faintness and thirst, and often vomits. If the condition develops he becomes listless and apathetic, and later unconscious.

OBJECTS OF TREATMENT.

The objects of treatment are to promote warmth of the body, to encourage a better circulation of blood in the brain, and to keep the patient's mind and body at rest.

TREATMENT.

(a) **Immediate** :—

1.—Arrest severe hæmorrhage if present.

2.—Lay the patient on his back on a rug, steadying and supporting any injured part. Place his head low and turned to one side.

3.—Loosen clothing about the neck, chest and waist, and ensure a free circulation of fresh air.

4.—Prevent aggravation of any injuries by temporary measures.

5.—Cover well with rugs or coats.

6.—Raise well the lower limbs.

7.—Apply smelling salts to the nose except in cases of head injury.

8.—Use encouraging words to the patient.

9.—Ensure freedom from excitement and worry.

10.—Do not discuss the patient's condition or injuries with others in his hearing.

11.—Remove the patient to shelter.

(*b*) **On arrival at shelter :—**

1.—Wrap the patient in blankets and apply hot water bottles to the sides of the body, between the legs and to the feet.

2.—If the patient is able to swallow, give freely hot, strong tea or coffee with plenty of sugar, except when injury to an internal organ is present or suspected. Avoid alcoholic stimulants.

3.—Examine for and treat all injuries, avoiding unnecessary handling or exposure of the injured parts.

Unless hæmorrhage from an internal organ is present or suspected, the removal of the patient from shelter to his home or to hospital may with advantage be delayed until the improving pulse, the return of colour and the disappearance of the beads of cold sweat from the face show that the condition has been effectively treated.

Chapter V.

DRESSINGS AND BANDAGES.

DRESSINGS.

A dressing is a covering applied to a wound or to an injured part.

The dressings used in First Aid are :—

1. Dry Dressing.—This is used to prevent contamination and to protect a wound, to promote healing, or to help in the application of correct pressure. The most reliable dressing for all wounds consists of a sterilised (germ-free) piece of gauze or lint stitched to a bandage ; this dressing is enclosed and sealed in a waxed paper covering ; this package is contained in an outer envelope on which are printed the directions for use.

If a sterilised dressing is not available the wound may be covered with a piece of clean gauze or lint or boracic lint.

In an emergency a perfectly clean handkerchief or piece of linen or clean unprinted paper, such as the inside of an envelope, may be used, but their use is only temporary until a sterilised dressing is available. Whenever possible, the improvised dressing should be soaked in an antiseptic solution (see page 106) and wrung dry.

2. Wet Dressings.

(a) A **cold compress** is used to ease pain, to lessen swelling, or to control internal bleeding. A clean handkerchief or piece of lint, four folds in thickness, is soaked in cold water, wrung out until it does not drip when held up, and applied to the affected part. It must be frequently changed in order to keep it cold and wet.

(b) A **hot compress** is used to ease pain. A piece of flannel or lint, four folds in thickness, is soaked in very hot water, wrung dry and applied to the affected part. As it is important to retain the heat as long as possible, it should be covered with a piece of jaconet, oiled silk or grease-proof paper larger than the compress. It must be renewed as soon as it cools.

All First Aid dressings, except the cold compress, should be **covered with cotton wool and kept in place by a bandage.**

BANDAGES.

Bandages form an important part of First Aid treatment, **the Triangular Bandage** being generally used.

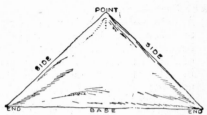

FIG. 12.—BANDAGE SPREAD OUT.

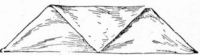

FIG. 13.—BANDAGE ONCE FOLDED.

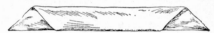

FIG. 14.—BROAD BANDAGE.

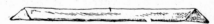

FIG. 15.—NARROW BANDAGE.

It may be applied

1. To retain splints or dressings in position.
2. To afford support to an injured part or as an arm sling.

3. To make pressure and so reduce or prevent swelling.

Triangular Bandages (Fig. 12) are made by cutting a piece of linen or calico about forty inches square diagonally into two pieces.

> **The broad bandage** is made by bringing the point down to the base (Fig. 13), and then folding into two (Fig. 14).

> **The narrow bandage** is made by folding the broad bandage once (Fig. 15).

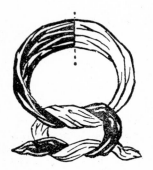 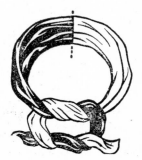

FIG. 16.—REEF KNOT.   FIG. 17.—GRANNY KNOT.

It is sometimes advisable to halve the size of the triangular bandage by bringing the two ends together before folding it into the broad or narrow bandage.

To secure the ends of a triangular bandage **Reef Knots** (Fig. 16) should be used. Granny knots (Fig. 17) are apt to slip and must be avoided. After the reef knot is completed, the ends of the bandage should be tucked in.

Bandages may be improvised from handkerchiefs, belts, straps, braces, neckties, or any piece of linen, calico, tape or cord that comes to hand.

Large arm sling (Fig. 18).—This supports the forearm and hand. Spread out a triangular bandage, put one end over the shoulder on the sound side, pass it round the neck so that it appears over the shoulder of the injured side, and let the other end hang down in front of the chest ; carry the point behind the elbow of the injured limb, and place the forearm over the middle of the bandage ; then carry the second end up to the first and tie them ; bring the point forward, and secure with two pins to the front of the bandage.

Small arm sling (Fig. 19).—This supports the wrist and hand but allows the elbow to hang freely. Place one end of a broad bandage over the shoulder on the sound side, pass it round the neck so that it appears over the shoulder of the injured side :

place the wrist over the middle of the bandage so that the front edge covers the base of the little finger; then bring the second end up to the first, and tie them.

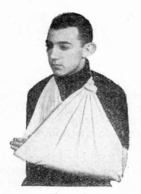 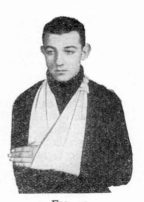

FIG. 18.
LARGE ARM SLING.

FIG. 19.
SMALL ARM SLING.

St. John Sling.—This keeps the hand well raised. (The following instructions apply in the case of an injury on the left side. When the injury is on the right side, substitute the word " left " for " right " and " right " for " left ").

(*a*) Place the patient's left forearm diagonally across the chest so that his fingers point towards the right shoulder and the palm rests on the breast-bone.

(*b*) Holding an unfolded bandage with its point in the right hand and one end in the left hand, lay the bandage over the left forearm with the point well beyond the elbow, and the end in the left hand on the right shoulder (Fig. 20).

(*c*) Whilst supporting the left elbow, tuck the base of the bandage well under the left hand and forearm and carry the lower end across the back to the right shoulder, allowing the point to hang loosely outwards ; tie the ends in the hollow above the right collar-bone.

(*d*) With your left hand hold open the side of the bandage lying on the left forearm, and with your right hand tuck the point well in between the left forearm and the side of the bandage which you are holding open.

(*e*) Carry the resulting fold round over the back of the arm, and firmly pin it to a part of the bandage running up the back (Figs. 21 and 22).

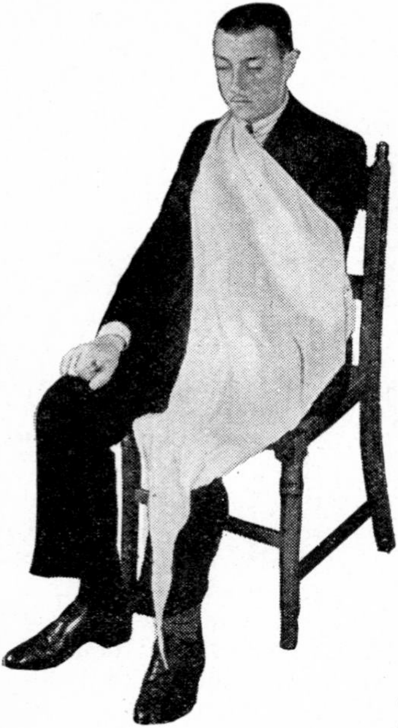

FIG. 20.

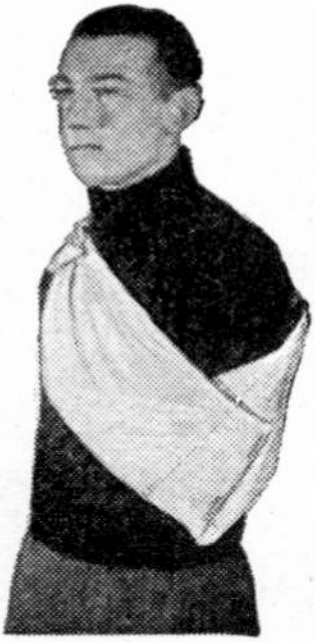

ST. JOHN SLING.

FIG. 21.

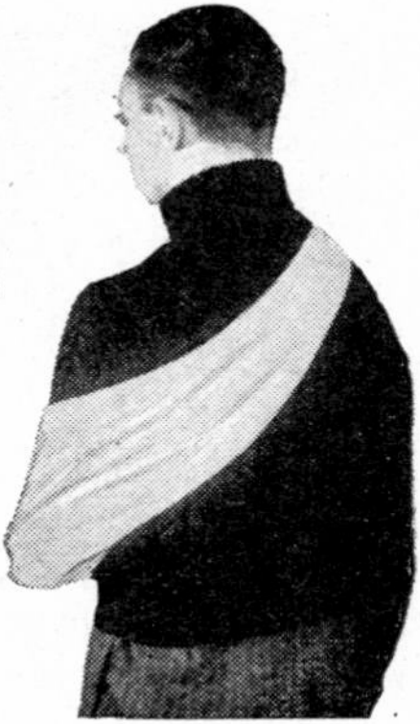

FIG. 22

Slings may be improvised in many simple ways, such as by pinning the sleeve to the clothing, turning up the lower edge of the coat, passing the hand inside the buttoned coat or waistcoat, etc.

APPLICATION OF BANDAGES.

For the Scalp (Fig. 23). Fold a hem inwards about 1½ inches deep along the base of a bandage ; place the bandage on the head so that the hem lies on the forehead **close down to the eyebrows,** and the point hangs down at the back ; carry the two ends round the head **above** the ears and tie them on the forehead so as to secure the lower border of the bandage ; steady the head with one hand and with the other draw the point of the bandage downwards ; then turn it up and pin it to the bandage on the top of the head.

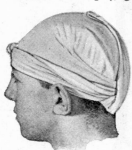

FIG. 23.
BANDAGE FOR SCALP.

For the Forehead, Side of the Head, Eye, Cheek, and for any part of the body that is round (as the arm or thigh, etc.), the narrow bandage should be used, its centre being placed over the dressing, and the ends carried round the head or limb, as the case may be, and tied.

For the Shoulder (Fig. 24). Place the centre of a bandage on the shoulder, with the point running

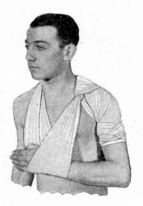

Fig. 24.
BANDAGE FOR SHOULDER.

up the side of the neck ; fold a hem inwards along the base ; carry the ends round the middle of the arm and tie them so as to secure the lower border of the bandage. Apply a small arm sling. Turn down the point of the first bandage over the knot of the sling, draw it tight and pin it.

For the Hip (Fig. 25). Tie a narrow bandage round the body above the haunch bones, with the

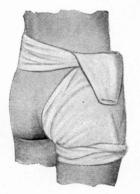

FIG. 25.
BANDAGE FOR HIP.

knot on the injured side. Carry the point of a second bandage under the first bandage and turn it down over the knot. Fold a hem inwards according to the size of the patient along the base

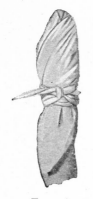

FIG. 26.
BANDAGE FOR HAND.

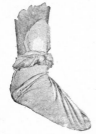

FIG. 27.
BANDAGE FOR FOOT.

of the second bandage, carry the ends round the thigh and tie them so as to secure the lower border of the bandage ; fix the point of the bandage with a safety pin.

For the Hand when the fingers are extended (Fig. 26). Fold a hem inwards along the base of a bandage ; place the injured surface on the bandage with the wrist on the hem and the fingers towards the point ; then bring the point over the wrist, pass the ends round the wrist, cross and tie them ; bring the point over the knot and pin it to the bandage over the hand. Apply a large arm sling.

For the Foot (Fig. 27). Place the foot on the centre of the bandage with the toes towards the point ; draw up the point over the instep, bring the ends forward and cross them; pass the ends round the ankle and tie them. Draw the point forward and pin it to the bandage over the instep.

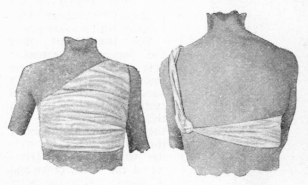

FIG. 28.   FIG. 29.

BANDAGE FOR CHEST.

(Front and back views.)

For the Front of the Chest (Figs. 28 and 29). Place the middle of the bandage over the dressing with the point over the shoulder on the same side; fold a three inch hem along the base of the bandage, carry the ends round the waist and tie them, leaving one end longer than the other ; then draw the point over the shoulder and tie it to the longer end.

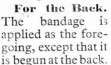

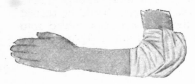

FIG. 30.
BANDAGE FOR ELBOW.

For the Back. The bandage is applied as the foregoing, except that it is begun at the back.

For the Elbow. (Fig. 30). Bend the elbow. Fold a narrow hem inwards along the base of a bandage ; lay the point on the back of the arm and the middle of the base on the back of the forearm ; cross the ends first in front of the elbow, then round the arm and tie them. Bring the point down and pin it.

For the Knee. (Fig. 31). Bend the knee. Fold a narrow hem inwards along the base of a bandage ; lay the point on the thigh and the middle of the base just below the knee-cap ; cross the ends first behind the knee, then round the thigh

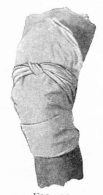

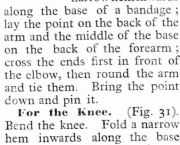

FIG. 31.
BANDAGE FOR KNEE.

and tie them. Bring the point down and pin it to the base.

When not in use, the triangular bandage should be folded narrow; the two ends should be turned to the centre, and the bandage then folded into four, reducing it to a packet about $6\frac{1}{2}$ inches by $3\frac{1}{2}$ inches.

CHAPTER VI.

FRACTURES.

Fracture is the term used when a bone is broken.

CAUSES OF FRACTURE.

1. Direct Violence.—When from a severe blow, impact of a bullet, crush of a wheel, etc., a bone breaks at the spot where the force is applied, the fracture is termed direct.

2. Indirect Violence.—When the bone breaks at some distance from the spot where the force is applied, the fracture is termed indirect. Alighting on the feet and fracturing either the thigh-bone or the bones of the leg, or falling on the hand and breaking either the radius or the collar-bone, are examples.

3. Muscular Action.—The knee-cap and the arm-bone are occasionally broken by a sudden violent contraction of the muscles attached to them.

Varieties of Fracture.

Fractures are classified in two ways :—

(A) According to the **condition of the tissues** adjacent to the bone :—

1. Simple.—The bone is broken with only slight injury to the surrounding tissues.

2. Compound.—The bone is broken and the skin and tissues are punctured or torn, thus allowing disease-producing germs to obtain access through the external wound to the seat of fracture. The fractured ends may protrude through the skin, or the wound may lead down to the fracture (for example, when a bone is broken by a bullet).

3. Complicated.—The bone is broken and in addition there is an injury to some internal organ (for example, the brain, spinal cord, lung, etc.) or to some important blood-vessel or nerve.

A fracture may be compound or complicated as the immediate result of the injury ; or a fracture, originally simple, may be converted into a compound or complicated fracture—

(a) by careless movement on the part of the patient, or

(b) by carelessness or ignorance on the part of anyone rendering aid.

(**B**) According to the **injury to the bone** itself :—

1. Comminuted.—The bone is broken into several pieces, and therefore requires special care in handling.

2. Greenstick.—In children, owing to the

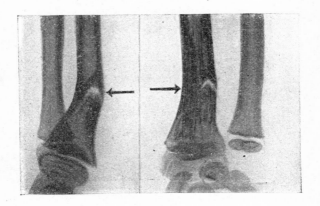

FIG. 32.
GREENSTICK FRACTURE OF RADIUS.
(Two Views.)

softer state of the bony tissues, a bone may bend and crack without breaking completely across (Fig. 32).

3. Impacted.—The broken ends of the bone are driven one into the other (Fig. 33).

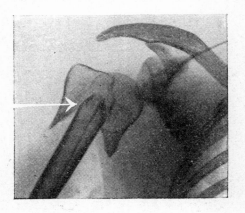

FIG. 33.

IMPACTED FRACTURE.

GENERAL SIGNS AND SYMPTOMS OF FRACTURE.

1. Pain at or near the seat of fracture.

2. Loss of power in the limb.

3. Swelling about the seat of fracture.—Swelling frequently renders it difficult to perceive other signs of fracture, and care must therefore be taken not to mistake a fracture for a less serious injury.

4. Deformity of the limb.—The limb assumes an unnatural position, and is mis-shapen at the seat of fracture. The contracting muscles may cause the broken ends of the bone to override, thereby producing shortening of the limb.

5. Irregularity of the bone.—If the bone is close to the skin the fracture may be felt.

6. Unnatural Mobility.—Movement may be noticed at the seat of fracture.

7. Crepitus, or bony grating, may be felt or heard when the broken ends move one upon the other.

The last two signs should be sought only by a doctor, and are absent in greenstick and impacted fractures.

In addition to the signs and symptoms the patient or the bystanders may be able to give the history of the injury ; and marks on the clothing or skin should be noted, as they may serve to locate the fracture. The snap of the bone may have been heard or felt.

angular
shortening

OBJECT OF TREATMENT.

The object of First Aid Treatment of Fractures is to guard against further injury or aggravation, especially to prevent a simple fracture from becoming compound or complicated.

GENERAL RULES FOR TREATMENT OF FRACTURE.

1. Attend to the fracture on the spot. No matter how crowded the thoroughfare, or how short the distance to a more convenient or comfortable place, no attempt must be made to move the patient until the limb has been rendered as immovable as practicable by splints or other means of restraint, unless life is in danger from some other cause.

2. When hæmorrhage accompanies a fracture it must be attended to first, and the wound covered by a clean dressing (see pages 1c6 and 107).

3. Steady and support the injured limb so that its further movement on the part of either the patient or the bystanders is prevented.

4. With great care and without using force place the limb in as natural a position as possible, and, if shortening is observed in the case of fracture of a bone of the lower limb, place one hand behind the heel and the other on the instep and pull evenly upon the foot (extension) until the limb regains a more normal length. When the

fix fracture above & below bones

limb is straightened, on no account let go until it is secured in position by splints, otherwise there is great danger of the fracture becoming compound or complicated. **Do not attempt extension in the case of a compound fracture when the bone protrudes.**

5. Apply splints, bandages and slings when necessary as follows :—

    (*a*) The splints must be firm, and long enough to keep the joints immediately above and below the fractured bone at rest. They should, if practicable, be well padded to fit accurately to the limb and be applied over the clothing. Ample width is very desirable in a splint. A splint may be improvised from a walking stick, umbrella, billiard cue, broom or brush handle, policeman's truncheon, rifle, folded coat, piece of wood, cardboard, paper firmly folded, a rolled-up map, or, in fact, **anything that is firm, long and wide enough to keep the joints immediately above and below the fractured bone at rest.** When the above appliances are not readily available, the upper limb, if fractured, may be tied to the trunk, and in all cases a fractured lower limb should be bandaged to its fellow.

(b) The bandages must be applied firmly, but not so tightly as to constrict the circulation of blood in the limb, thereby producing congestion in the extremity. When the patient is in the recumbent position, double the bandage over the end of a splint to pass it under the trunk or lower limb, using the natural hollows of the body (the neck, loins, knees and just above the heels). Avoid jarring the patient whilst working them into their correct position. As a general rule :—

For the trunk the broad bandage should be used. Pass it once round the trunk and fasten it by tying the ends (or with two or three safety pins) on the side opposite to the fracture, but if to secure a splint for a broken thigh, tie or fasten the ends over the splint.

For the limbs the narrow bandage should be used. Pass it twice round the limb, and tie the ends over the outer splint ; or it may be more convenient to double the bandage at the centre, pass it under the limb, bring the loop over the limb, pass both ends of the bandage through it in opposite directions, and tie them over the outer splint (Loop bandage, Fig. 34). If sufficient bandages are not available, the splints in fractures of the limbs may be secured by strips of adhesive plaster.

When applying bandages near a fracture the upper one should be secured first. When securing an improvised round splint, an extra turn of the bandage should be made round the splint to hold it in position.

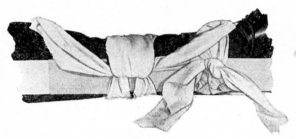

FIG. 34.—LOOP BANDAGE.

(c) Slings, when necessary, should be applied as described in Chapter V.

In all doubtful cases treat as a fracture.

SPECIAL FRACTURES.

Fracture of the Skull.—A fracture of the upper part is usually caused by direct violence—for example, a blow on the head. A fracture of the base is caused by indirect violence, through a fall on the head, a fall on the feet or lower part of the spine, or a severe blow on the lower jaw. *If the upper part is fractured,* the signs are swelling, irregularity, and frequently insensibility, either immediate or coming on gradually. *If the base is fractured,* insensibility may come on immediately, blood or fluid may issue from the ear channel (see page 139), escape from the nose, or it may pass down to the stomach, whence it may be vomited; the fracture may involve the orbit, causing a blood-shot eye. Injury to the brain is the great danger attending a fracture of the skull.

TREATMENT.

See "Concussion and Compression of the Brain," page 163.

Fracture of the Lower Jaw.—Pain, loss of power (inability to speak and to move the jaw freely), irregularity of the teeth, crepitus and bleeding from the gum are the usual signs and symptoms.

TREATMENT.

1.—Place the palm of the hand below the injured bone and press it gently against the upper jaw.

2.—Apply the centre of a narrow bandage under the chin, carry both ends upwards and tie above the forehead.

3.—Apply the centre of a narrow bandage in front of the chin, carry both ends backwards and tie at the back of the neck (Figs. 35 and 36).

4.—Tie the ends of both bandages together.

5.—If the patient shows any indication of being about to vomit, remove bandages immediately, turn head to the sound side and support the jaw with the palm of the hand. Re-apply bandages when vomiting has completely ceased.

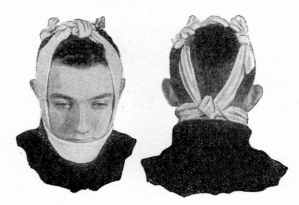

FIG. 35.   FIG. 36.
BANDAGE FOR FRACTURE OF LOWER JAW.

Fracture of the Spine.—The vertebral column may be broken either by direct or indirect violence. The fall of a heavy weight upon the back, and falling from a height on the back across a bar or upon an uneven surface are examples of direct violence ; and a fall on the head, causing a broken neck, is an example of indirect violence (see Fig. 37).

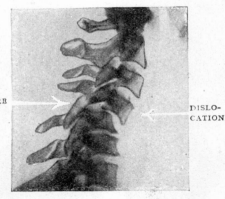

FRACTURE

DISLO-
CATION

FIG. 37.

FRACTURE OF THE SPINE
(CERVICAL), WITH DISLOCATION.

What is commonly regarded as a broken back consists of a fracture of one or more of the vertebræ with displacement of the fragments, whereby the spinal cord and the nerves issuing from it may be injured, causing complete or partial loss of power and sensation (paralysis) in all parts of the body below the seat of fracture. Pain is present at the seat of injury and shock may be severe.

RULES FOR TREATMENT IN ALL CASES OF SPINAL INJURY.

1.—Immediately warn the patient to lie still.

2.—Apply a bandage in the manner of the figure 8 round ankles and feet, the knot being tied under the soles of the feet. Apply broad bandages round the knees and round the thighs.

3.—If a doctor is not readily available, remove the patient to shelter as follows :—

TRANSPORT.

A. If the patient is **unconscious** or if the situation of the injury is not clearly defined, the patient should be carried in the **face-upwards** (supine) position.

B. (i) If the patient is **conscious** but cannot move his arms or legs of his own accord or has no sensation in them, suspect a fracture in the **cervical region (a** broken neck) and transport him **face-**

C❉

upwards with pads 4 inches thick, one under the neck and one on each side of the neck to prevent movements of the head and neck.

(ii) If the patient is **conscious** but cannot move one or both legs of his own accord or has no sensation in them, **while retaining the use of his arms,** suspect a fracture in the **thoracic or lumbar region** and transport the patient in the **face-downwards** (prone) position.

To Transport a Case of Spinal Injury in the Face-Upwards Position.

1.—If the patient is found lying in any position except on the back, with great care and with all the assistance available, slowly and evenly roll him on to his back. If the patient is unconscious, ensure that breathing does not become obstructed by the tongue (see page 141).

2.—Lay a blanket or rug folded smoothly on a shutter, door or board of at least the same length and width as the patient. Failing this, the entire bed of a stretcher must be stiffened, preferably with a series of short transverse boards.

3.—Without moving the patient, pass looped broad bandages from alternate sides under the natural hollows of the body (the neck, loins and knees); without jerking, work them into position under (*a*) the head, (*b*) shoulder-blades, (*c*) buttocks, (*d*) thighs and (*e*) calves.

4.—Pass long poles, pitch-fork handles, etc., through the loops on each side. Tie the free ends of the bandages over the poles.

5.—Place the patient on the stretcher as follows :—

    (*a*) *If five bearers are available*, two should stand on each side of the patient facing one another, and, on the word of command being given, grasp the poles firmly, with hands well apart, and slowly and evenly raise the patient sufficiently high to enable the fifth bearer to push the stretcher under.

    (*b*) *If only four bearers are available*, they should lift the patient as in (*a*) above, and then move with short side paces till the patient is directly over the stretcher, care having been taken to place the foot of the stretcher as close to the head of the patient as convenient before proceeding to lift.

    (*c*) *If only three bearers are available*, one should stand on each side of the patient facing one another. On the word of command being given, they stoop down and grasp the poles firmly, the hands well apart, opposite shoulders and hips ; the third bearer faces the feet and firmly grips the end of each pole. They then slowly and evenly raise the patient and move with short paces till the patient is directly over the stretcher, care having been taken to place the foot of the stretcher as close to the head of the patient as convenient before proceeding to lift.

6.—On reaching shelter nothing further is to be done until the arrival of a doctor.

To Transport a Case of Spinal Injury in the Face-Downwards Position.

1. Prepare the stretcher, **which must not be boarded,** and arrange blankets as on page 208 (Figs. 91 and 92).

2.—Fold and roll two blankets. The rolls must be firm and as wide as the stretcher.

3.—With great care and using all the assistance available, roll and support the patient on his side.

4.—Turn the stretcher on to its side, close to the front of the patient's body; place the rolled blankets in position, one across the front of the patient's shoulders and the other across the front of his hips (Fig. 38).

5.—Holding the stretcher in close contact with the patients' body, carefully turn the stretcher

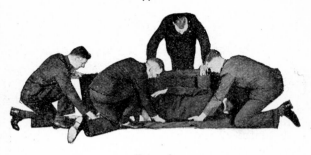

FIG. 38.
TURNING A CASE OF SPINAL INJURY.

and patient, as one, into the correct position for
carrying (Fig. 39). The turning of the patient on
to his face may be assisted by the bearers pulling
on the edge of the blanket under him.

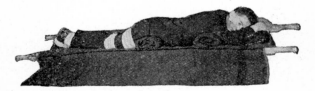

FIG. 39.
CASE TURNED.

6.—Turn the patient's head slightly to one side and support it on a pillow.

7.—On reaching shelter nothing further must be done until the arrival of a doctor.

Fractured Ribs.—The ribs usually fractured are the sixth, seventh, eighth, or ninth, and generally the fracture is midway between the breast-bone and the spine. The fracture may be caused by indirect violence, driving the fractured ends of the bone outwards, or by direct violence, driving the fractured ends of the bone inwards and sometimes injuring the lungs or other internal organ. If the lower ribs on the right side are broken, the liver may be injured, and a fracture of the lower left ribs may wound the spleen. Evidence of the fracture is afforded by a sharp cutting pain, especially on attempting to take a deep breath, and by short and shallow breathing. If the lungs are injured blood, frothy and bright red, may be coughed up and expectorated. If the liver or spleen is wounded hæmorrhage may occur internally (see page 137).

TREATMENT.

(a) *Simple fracture.*—*When the fracture is not complicated by an injury to an internal organ :—*

1.—Apply two broad bandages round the chest firmly enough to afford support, with the centre of the first immediately above and that of the second immediately below the seat of the pain. The lower bandage should overlap the upper to half its extent. The knots are to be tied rather to

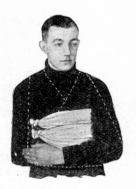

FIG. 40.
BANDAGE FOR SIMPLE
FRACTURE OF RIBS.

the front on the opposite side of the body. Another plan is to apply a strong towel, folded about eight inches wide, firmly round the chest, securing it with three or four safety pins.

2.—Place the arm on the injured side in a large sling (Fig. 40):

(b) Complicated fracture.—When an internal organ is injured :—

    1.—Do not apply bandages round the chest.

    2.—Lay the patient down with the body inclined toward the injured side, and supported in that position.

    3.—Loosen the clothing, give ice to suck, and apply a cold compress to the seat of injury.

    4.—Treat as for hæmorrhage from an internal organ (see page 137).

    5.—Place the arm on the injured side in a large sling.

Fracture of the Breast-bone.—

When this fracture can be felt or is suspected, undo all tight clothing about the chest. Place the patient on his back in the most comfortable position and remove him to shelter.

Fracture of the Collar-bone.—This fracture is frequently caused by a fall on the hand or shoulder. The arm on the injured side is partially helpless, and the patient usually supports it at the elbow with his hand, and inclines his head towards the injured side. The fractured ends can generally be felt to overlap, the outer fragment being the lower. The general signs and symptoms of fracture are present.

TREATMENT.

1.—Remove the coat and as much more of the clothing as is expedient. Unfasten a man's brace on the injured side.

2.—Place in the armpit a pad, about two inches thick, two inches broad and four inches across, which will act as a fulcrum.

3.—Apply a St. John sling.

4.—Secure the injured limb firmly to the side by a broad bandage passed round the elbow and trunk, so as to lever out and draw back the shoulder (Fig. 41).

5.—Ascertain that the pulse is present at the wrist ; if it is not, relax the bandage around the body.

6.—Tighten the sling.

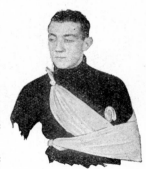

FIG. 41.
BANDAGE FOR SIMPLE
FRACTURE OF COLLAR-BONE.

Fracture of the Shoulder-blade is very rare.

TREATMENT.

Apply the centre of a broad bandage in the armpit of the injured side, cross the ends over the uninjured shoulder and tie them in the armpit (Fig. 42). Support the injured limb in a St. John sling.

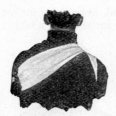

FIG. 42.
BANDAGE FOR SIMPLE FRACTURE OF SHOULDER BLADE.

Fracture of the Arm.— The bone may be broken :— (*a*) close to the shoulder ; (*b*) near the middle of the shaft ; (*c*) close to or involving the elbow-joint.

TREATMENT.

(*a*) *When the Fracture is close to the Shoulder*—

1.—Apply a broad bandage with its upper border level with the top of the shoulder ; pass it round the limb and body and tie it on the opposite side under the armpit.

2.—Apply a small arm sling.

(b) When the Fracture is near the Middle of the Shaft—

1.—Place the forearm across the chest at a right angle to the arm.

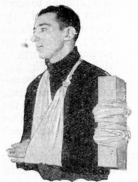

2.—Apply a small arm sling.

3.—Apply splints, reaching from the shoulder to the elbow, on the front, back and outer side of the arm in its present position.

4.—Secure the splints by bandages above and below the fracture (Fig. 43).

If splints are not available, secure the arm to the side by two broad bandages.

FIG. 43.
TREATMENT OF
FRACTURE OF ARM.

(c) When the fracture, whether of the arm or forearm, involves the elbow-joint.—

This fracture is attended with much swelling, and it is difficult to ascertain the exact nature of the injury.

1.—Take two splints, one long enough to reach from the arm-pit to below the elbow, the other long enough to reach from beyond the elbow to the finger tips ; tie them together to form a right angle (Fig. 44).

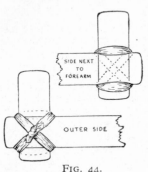

SIDE NEXT TO FOREARM

OUTER SIDE

FIG. 44.
ANGULAR SPLINT.

2.—Apply the angular splint so made on the side of the flexed limb that shows the less injury.

3.—Secure the splint by bandages (*a*) round the arm (*b*) round the forearm, and (*c*) a third as a figure of 8 round the hand and wrist.

4.—Apply a small arm sling.

5.—Apply a cold compress over the fracture to reduce the swelling.

Fracture of the Forearm.—When both bones are broken, the general signs and symptoms of fracture are usually present. When one of the bones only is broken the signs and symptoms are as a rule pain, loss of power, swelling, and irregularity.

An impacted fracture of the Radius just above the wrist is a common result of a fall on the hand.

TREATMENT.

This is the same, whether the fracture involves one bone or both.

1.—Place the forearm at a right angle to the arm, across the chest, keeping the thumb uppermost, and the palm of the hand towards the body.

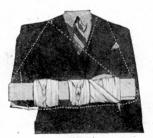

FIG. 45.

TREATMENT OF FRACTURE OF FOREARM.

2.—Apply splints on the front and back of the forearm from the elbow to the fingers.

3.—Apply 2 bandages, embracing both splints; one is placed above the fracture, and the other round the wrist first and completed as a figure of 8 round the hand and wrist (Fig. 45).

4.—Apply a large arm sling.

Fracture of the bones of the Hand or Fingers—Crushed Hand.

TREATMENT.

1.—Apply a carefully padded splint to the front of the hand, reaching from the middle of the forearm to beyond the tips of the fingers.

2.—To secure the splint apply a bandage, crossed in the manner of the figure 8, to the hand and wrist and a second bandage round the forearm (Fig. 46).

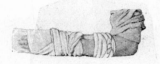

FIG. 46.
TREATMENT OF CRUSHED
HAND.

3.—Apply a large arm sling.

Fracture of the Pelvis.—When, after a severe injury in the neighbourhood of the haunch-bones there is no sign of damage to the lower limbs, but the patient is unable to stand or even to move the lower limbs without great difficulty and pain, a fracture of the pelvis may be assumed to have occurred. The blood-vessels and organs within the pelvis, especially the bladder, are in danger of being injured.

TREATMENT.

1.—Lay the patient in whatever position is found to give the greatest ease, and flex or straighten the lower limbs as the patient desires.

2.—Apply a broad bandage round the pelvis, in line with the hip joints, tight enough to support the parts, but not so tight as to press the broken bone further inwards.

3.—Apply a bandage as a figure of 8 round ankles and feet and a broad bandage round both knees.

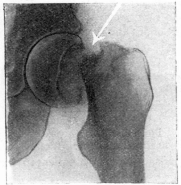

FIG. 47.
FRACTURE OF NECK OF FEMUR.

Fracture of the Thigh-bone. — The thigh-bone may be broken at its neck, anywhere in the shaft or close to the knee. All the general signs and symptoms of fracture are usually present and a prominent sign is the position of the foot, which lies on its outer side. Shortening may vary from one-half to three inches. A fracture at the neck (Fig. 47) is likely to occur in old people from a very slight cause, and is often difficult to distinguish from a severe bruise of the hip ; but it may be assumed that when, after an injury near the hip-joint, the patient cannot, when lying on the back, raise the heel from the ground, the bone is broken. The danger from shock is great.

TREATMENT.

1.—Steady the limb by holding the ankle and foot. Gently draw down the foot, bringing it into line with its fellow, and apply a bandage as a figure of 8 round the ankles and feet. (Bandage A.)

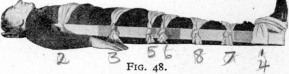

FIG. 48.

TREATMENT OF FRACTURE OF THIGH-BONE.

2.—Pass seven bandages under the patient in the following order :—

The chest, just below the armpits (B).

The pelvis, in line with the hip joints (C).

Both ankles and feet (D). This covers bandage A.

Both thighs, above the fracture (E).

Both thighs, below the fracture (F).

Both legs (G).

Both knees (H) (a **broad** bandage).

3.—Place a splint along the injured side of the patient from the armpit to just beyond the foot.

4.—Secure the splint by tying the bandages in the same order. All the bandages should be tied over the splint except D, which should be applied as a figure of 8 and tied under the soles of the feet (Fig. 48).

FIG. 49.

FRACTURE OF KNEE-CAP.

Fracture of the Knee-cap.— The knee-cap may be broken by direct violence, but more frequently it is broken by muscular action, as follows :—When the foot slips, in the attempt to prevent a fall, the muscles in the front of the thigh act with such force as to snap the knee-cap in two (Fig. 49).

Pain, loss of power (the limb will be quite helpless), irregularity (a gap may be felt between the broken fragments of bone) and swelling accompany this injury.

TREATMENT.

1.—Lay the patient on his back, raise well and support the head and shoulders, straighten and raise the limb.

2.—Apply a splint along the back of the limb, reaching from the buttock to beyond the heel. The splint must be well padded under the natural hollow of the leg so as to raise the heel from the splint.

3.—Secure the splint by bandages round the thigh (A), and leg (B) (Fig. 50).

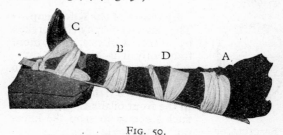

FIG. 50.
TREATMENT OF FRACTURE OF KNEE-CAP.

4.—Secure the foot by a double figure of 8 bandage round splint, ankle, foot and splint, tying on top of the splint below the foot (C).

5.—Support the foot well off the ground by a pillow, roll of clothing or rugs.

6.—Apply a narrow bandage with its centre immediately above the knee-cap, cross the ends behind over the splint, pass them again to the front of the limb just below the knee-cap and tie them (D).

7.—Apply a cold compress over the fracture to lessen swelling of the joint.

Fracture of the Leg.—One or both of the bones may be broken. When both bones are broken all the general signs of fracture are usually present, but when one bone only is broken deformity is not always noticeable. A fracture of the fibula three or four inches above its lower end is frequently mistaken for a sprain and sometimes for a dislocation of the ankle.

TREATMENT.

1.—Steady the limb by holding the ankle and foot.

2.—Draw the foot into its natural position, and do not let go until the splints have been fixed.

3.—Apply splints on the outer and inner sides of the leg, reaching from above the knee to beyond the foot. If only one splint is available place it on the outer side.

4.—Secure the splints by bandages (A) above, (B) below the fracture, (C) immediately above the knee, (D) round ankles and feet as a figure of 8, (E) a broad bandage round both knees (Fig. 51).

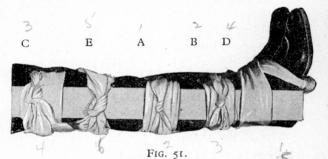

FIG. 51.

TREATMENT OF FRACTURE OF LEG.

When single-handed, after extending the limb tie ankles and feet together, dispense with the inner splint, and pass the bandages round both limbs in the order shown in Fig. 51.

When no splint is available the feet, ankles, knees and thighs should be tied together.

Fracture of the bones of the Foot or Toes— Crushed Foot.

This injury is commonly caused by the passage of a heavy weight over the foot, and may be recognised by pain, swelling, and loss of power.

TREATMENT.

1.—Remove the boot and stocking.

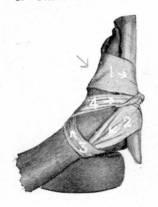

FIG. 52.

TREATMENT OF CRUSHED FOOT.

2.—Apply a carefully padded splint to the sole of the foot, reaching from the heel to the toes.

3.—Apply the centre of a narrow bandage over the instep, crossing it after the manner of the figure 8 as shown in Fig. 52, tying it off on the splint.

4.—Support the foot in a slightly raised position.

CHAPTER VII.

INJURIES TO JOINTS AND MUSCLES.

DISLOCATIONS.

A dislocation is the displacement of one or more of the bones at a joint.

The joints most frequently dislocated are those of the shoulder, elbow, thumb, fingers, and lower jaw.

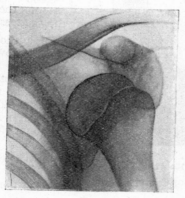

FIG. 53.
DISLOCATION OF SHOULDER.

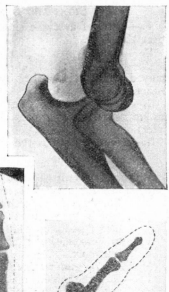

FIG. 54.

DISLOCATION OF
ELBOW.

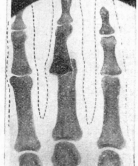

FIG. 55. (Back View.)   FIG. 56. (Side View.)
DISLOCATION OF FINGER.

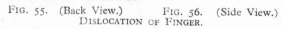

Signs and Symptoms.

1.—Pain of a severe sickening character at or near the joint.

2.—Loss of power in the limb.

3.—Fixity of the joint.—The limb cannot be moved at the joint either by the patient or First-Aider.

4.—Deformity of the limb.—The limb assumes an unnatural position, and is mis-shapen at the joint.

5.—Swelling about the joint.

Treatment.

Make no attempt to reduce a dislocation.

(a) *When the accident occurs out of doors—*
> Steady and support the limb in the position which gives most ease to the patient, using padding where necessary in order to lessen the effects of jolting during transport.

(b) *When the patient is indoors—*
> 1.—Rest the patient on a couch or bed in the position which gives most ease.
>
> 2.—If the pain is severe, expose the injured part and apply a cold compress.
>
> 3.—When cold ceases to give comfort apply a hot compress.

DISPLACED CARTILAGES.

In sudden wrenches of the knee such as are met with in football and other games or slipping on a step the semi-lunar cartilages may be displaced or torn.

The signs (except for deformity), symptoms and treatment are the same as those of a dislocation.

SPRAINS.

When, by a sudden wrench or twist, *the ligaments and the parts around a joint* are stretched or torn the joint is said to be sprained.

SIGNS AND SYMPTOMS.

1.—Pain at the joint.

2.—Inability to use the joint without increasing the pain.

3.—Swelling and, later, discoloration.

TREATMENT.

1.—Place the limb in the most comfortable position and prevent any movement.

2.—Expose the joint and apply a firm bandage.

3.—Wet the bandage with cold water and keep it wet.

4.—When this ceases to give relief, take the bandage off and re-apply it.

In all doubtful cases treat as a fracture.

D

STRAINS AND RUPTURED MUSCLES.

When, during severe exertion, *muscles or tendons* are over-stretched they are said to be strained ; or, if they are actually torn, they are described as ruptured.

A so-called strain in the groin (hernia) is an injury of a totally different nature (see page 183).

Signs and Symptoms.

1.—A sudden sharp pain at the seat of injury.

2.—When the muscles of a limb are strained they may swell and cause severe cramp.

3.—Further exertion is difficult or impossible ; for example, if the strain has occurred in the back the patient may be unable to stand upright.

Treatment.

1.—Place the patient in the most comfortable position, and afford support to the injured part.

2.—Apply a hot compress.

CHAPTER VIII.

THE CIRCULATION OF THE BLOOD.

The organs concerned in the circulation of the blood are the **Heart**, the **Arteries**, the **Capillaries** and the **Veins**.

The **Heart** is a muscular organ which acts like a pump. It is situated in the chest behind the breast-bone and rib cartilages, between the lungs and immediately above the diaphragm; it lies obliquely with a quarter of its bulk to the right, and the remaining three-quarters to the left of the middle line of the body. Its beat may be felt just below and to the inner side of the left nipple. The heart has four cavities, two on either side of a central partition. The two upper cavities are named the **right and left auricles**, the two lower the **right and left ventricles**.

The heart contracts in adults at an average rate of seventy-two times a minute, but the rate increases as the position is changed from the lying to the sitting, and, still more, to the standing position; hence the importance of considering the patient's position in cases of bleeding. At every contraction

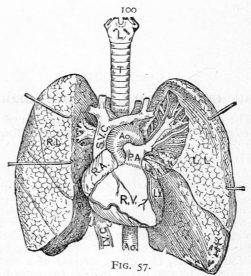

FIG. 57.

DIAGRAM OF HEART, LUNGS AND AIR-PASSAGES.

L. Larynx (voice box) ; T. Trachea (wind pipe) ; R.L. Right Lung ; L.L. Left Lung (the lungs are drawn back to expose the heart and blood vessels) ; R.A. Right Auricle ; L.A. Left Auricle ; R.V. Right Ventricle ; L.V. Left Ventricle ; P.A. Pulmonary Artery ; Ao. Aorta ; S.V.C. Superior vena cava (the large vein carrying blood from the upper part of the body to the heart) ; I.V.C. Inferior vena cava (the large vein carrying blood from the lower part of the body to the heart). The four pulmonary veins cannot be shown in the diagram.

of the left ventricle blood is forced into the **arteries,** which have a large amount of elastic tissue in their walls, and causes them to dilate, producing the regular expansion known as the **pulse,** which, corresponding with each beat of the heart, may be felt wherever the finger can be placed on an artery as it lies over a bone. (See pages 121 and 188.)

In the general (systemic) circulation the purified bright red blood in the left ventricle of the heart is driven into the main artery of the body (Aorta). The blood is propelled forward by the force of the contractions of the heart, and by the recoil of the elastic walls of the arteries, which have been dilated by the blood at each beat of the heart. From the aorta, branch-arteries are given off to all parts of the body. These arteries divide and sub-divide, becoming smaller and smaller, and terminate in very thin walled vessels (**capillaries**). Through these thin walls of the capillaries, an interchange of gases and fluids takes place. The blood gives off oxygen gas and nourishment to the tissues and organs of the body, and takes up from them carbonic acid gas and waste matters. The presence of these impurities changes the colour of the blood from bright to dark red. The capillaries unite to form small **veins,** and these join with other veins, becoming larger and larger until they have all united to form two large veins (Venæ Cavæ), which enter the right auricle of the heart. The blood is helped onwards in the

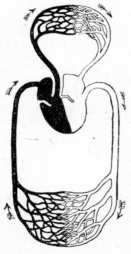

Explanation.—In the middle of the diagram is the heart with its four chambers. Above the heart is shown the lung (pulmonary) circulation. The lower part represents the general (systemic) circulation. Vessels containing impure (venous) blood are shown black, while those containing pure (arterial) blood are shown white. The connecting vessels represent the capillaries. The arrows show the direction of the flow of blood.

FIG. 58.

DIAGRAM OF THE CIRCU-LATION OF THE BLOOD.

veins by the suction action of the heart, which dilates after being emptied at each contraction. The veins are provided at frequent intervals with valves, which allow the blood to flow forward and close to prevent any backward flow.

From the right auricle of the heart the blood passes into the right ventricle ; and the contraction of the ventricle forces it into the **Pulmonary Artery,** which carries it to the lungs. This artery also divides into capillaries in the lungs so that an interchange of gases takes place between the air and the blood. Here it gives off its carbonic acid gas and impurities and takes up oxygen, thus becoming purified and bright red in colour. The capillaries unite to form the pulmonary veins which convey the blood to the left auricle of the heart, whence it passes to the left ventricle, and so completes the round of the circulation.

CHAPTER IX.

WOUNDS AND HÆMORRHAGE.

A **Wound** is a break in the continuity of the tissues of the body which permits the escape of blood and the entrance of disease-producing germs or other injurious agents.

Wounds may be classified as follows :—

1.—Incised wounds, which are caused by a sharp instrument, such as a razor, and bleed freely, as the blood vessels are " clean cut."

2.—Lacerated wounds, which have torn and irregular edges. They are caused by such things as machinery, a piece of shell or the claws of an animal. As the blood vessels are torn through, lacerated wounds bleed less freely than incised wounds, and the bleeding may be delayed for a time.

3.—Contused wounds, which are accompanied by bruising of the tissues, and are caused by a direct blow by some blunt instrument or by crushing.

4.—Punctured wounds, which have comparatively small openings, but may be very deep and are caused by a stab from any sharp-pointed instrument, as a needle, knife or bayonet.

Gun-shot wounds come under one or more of the above headings.

Hæmorrhage, or bleeding, is of three kinds :—
1. Arterial. 2. Capillary. 3. Venous.

ARTERIAL HÆMORRHAGE.

1.—Blood from an artery is bright red.

2.—If the wounded artery is near the skin the blood spurts out in jets corresponding with the pulsation of the heart.

3.—Blood issues from the side of the wound nearer to the heart.

CAPILLARY HÆMORRHAGE.

1.—The blood is red.

2.—It may flow briskly in a continuous stream or merely ooze from all parts of the wound.

VENOUS HÆMORRHAGE.

1.—Blood from a vein is dark red.

2.—It flows in a steady, continuous stream.

3.—It issues from the side of the wound further from the heart.

D*

OBJECTS OF TREATMENT OF WOUNDS.

**The objects of First Aid treatment of wounds
are :—**

1.—**To stop the bleeding.** As a clot of blood
is Nature's method of stopping bleeding, it should
never be disturbed when present over a wound.
A blood clot serves the double purpose of keeping
blood in and germs out.

2.—**To lessen the effects of shock.**

3.—**To prevent contamination** (sepsis) caused
by the entrance of minute living organisms called
germs, which are present in the air, in water, and
on all surrounding objects, such as the hands,
clothes, etc.

It is very easy to introduce germs into a wound,
however small :—

    (a) by unnecessarily touching it or the dressing
        which is to be applied unless the hands are
        perfectly clean and have been made sterile
        by the application of an **antiseptic.**
        An antiseptic is a chemical substance which
        has the power of restraining the development
        of germs. Antiseptics which do not stain,
        burn or irritate and which are not
        poisonous, are preferable. If these are
        not available, normal saline solution (one

teaspoonful of salt to a pint of sterile water), may be used;

(b) by washing it with water which has not been rendered sterile by being boiled and allowed to cool, or by the addition of an antiseptic;

(c) by leaving it exposed to the air;

(d) by the application of sticking plaster or ointment.

To ensure as far as possible the cleanliness of all dressings used :—

1.—Spread out a clean handkerchief, triangular bandage or towel and on it place all the necessary material.

2 (a).—If using a sterilised dressing remove the outer envelope, sterilise the fingers and open the inner package ; remove the dressing, taking care to expose it as little as possible to the air, and avoid fingering the surface of the dressing. After sterilising the fingers care **must** be taken not to handle anything which is not clean.

(b).—If a sterilised dressing is not available, sterilise the fingers, cut a piece of clean gauze, lint or boracic lint to the required size and apply to the wound. Avoid touching the side of the dressing which is placed next to the wound.

3.—After the dressing is completed, again sterilise the fingers and replace the unused dressings in a clean container.

GENERAL RULES FOR TREATMENT OF A WOUND ACCOMPANIED BY ARTERIAL HÆMORRHAGE.

1.—Place the patient in a suitable position, bearing in mind that blood escapes with less force when the patient sits, and still less when he lies down.

2.—Elevate the bleeding part, except in the case of a fractured limb.

3.—Expose the wound, removing only whatever clothing may be necessary.

4.—Immediately apply pressure with the thumb or fingers (digital pressure), either—

(a).—**directly on the bleeding spot** (direct digital pressure). Direct pressure must not be made over a fracture or foreign body ; or

(b).—if the wound is large, or if a foreign body or a fracture is suspected, on a point, known as **the pressure point,** as near as possible to the wound on the heart side where the artery can be pressed against the underlying bone (indirect digital pressure). When making indirect digital pressure, avoid crooking the thumb or fingers and digging the tips into the part. The nearest pressure point is chosen in order to avoid cutting off the circulation from as much of the part as possible, but sometimes it is necessary to apply pressure still nearer to the heart. (See pages 113—126.)

5.—As soon as practicable substitute for digital pressure a **pad and bandage** or if necessary a **tourniquet** on the pressure point while the wound is being examined and treated.

6.—**Remove any foreign bodies**, such as broken glass, bits of clothing, hair, which can be seen lying loose in the wound ; do not search for foreign bodies which cannot be seen.

7.—**If the wound is obviously dirty, and medical aid cannot be procured, wash away as much of the dirt as possible** by gently pouring sterilised water over it freely, notwithstanding the fact that wounds heal best if kept dry. **Never wash the surrounding parts towards a wound.**

8.—**Apply an antiseptic all over the wound and the surrounding skin, and cover with a dry dressing.**

9.—**Cover the dressing** with cotton wool, lint or other soft material.

10.—Apply a bandage over the dressing firmly ; but if the presence of a foreign body or fracture is suspected apply it lightly.

11.—Relax indirect pressure and note whether bleeding has ceased. If it has, leave the relaxed pad and bandage or tourniquet in position ; if it has not, re-apply indirect pressure. As prolonged maintenance of indirect pressure may cause dangerous congestion in the limb, prompt steps to obtain medical aid are extremely necessary. If it is not obtainable within twenty minutes, at the end of that time again relax indirect pressure and note whether bleeding recurs. If necessary, re-apply indirect pressure and repeat these steps at intervals of twenty minutes until medical aid is obtained.

12.—Afford support to the injured part.

IMPROVISATION OF A TOURNIQUET.

(*a*) Apply a firm pad on the pressure point.

(*b*) Encircle the limb by a narrow bandage or strap with its centre over the pad, and tie the ends in a half knot on the opposite side.

(*c*) Lay a short, strong stick or other similar object on the half knot, and over it tie a reef knot.

(*d*) Twist the stick to tighten the bandage, thereby pressing the pad upon the artery and arresting the flow of blood.

(*e*) Lock the stick in position by the ends of the bandage already applied, or by another bandage passed round the stick and limb.

The pad of the tourniquet must be accurately placed upon the pressure point so as completely to compress the artery; otherwise arterial blood will be allowed to pass along the limb, and the veins, being compressed by the tourniquet, will not allow the blood to return through them to the heart, and the result will be dangerous swelling and congestion.

Should a suitable pad not be at hand, a knot may be made in the centre of the bandage, and when available, a stone, cork, etc., enclosed in it to give it firmness and bulk. See that the bulging and not the flat side of the knot is on the pressure point.

The use of elastic bandages, except when part of a limb is cut or torn off, is to be rigorously avoided, as it stops the return flow of blood through the veins.

St. John Tourniquet.

A very useful form of tourniquet is known as the " St. John " (Fig. 59), which consists of a piece of webbing two inches wide (**B**), provided with a buckle (**D**), pad (**A**) and twister (**C**) over the pad,

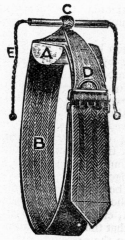

FIG. 59.
ST. JOHN TOURNIQUET.

First place the pad on the pressure point, pass the band round the limb and, both while and after buckling firmly, ensure that the pad is in correct position ; then apply sufficient pressure with the twister to arrest hæmorrhage, keeping the twister as near the centre of the pad as possible. Finally secure the twister by the string (**E**) passing through it, which should be tied to the **D** of the buckle, or may be temporarily secured by passing it between the webbing and the part of the buckle on which the spikes rest.

(Students practising arrest of arterial hæmorrhage in the limbs should feel the pulse of the radial or posterior tibial, artery, as the case may be, to note when the flow of blood in the artery stops, and should then immediately relax the pressure made on the artery. In this way the importance of the accurate application of pressure will be realised, and the amount of force necessary will be ascertained.)

THE COURSE OF THE MAIN ARTERIES, AND THE ARREST OF ARTERIAL HÆMORRHAGE.

(The numbers of the pressure points in the text refer to those on the Frontispiece.)

THE LARGE ARTERIES WITHIN THE CHEST AND ABDOMEN.

The Aorta is the central or trunk artery of the body. Commencing at the left ventricle, it forms an arch behind the upper part of the breast-bone. From the arch are given off the large branches which carry the blood to either side of the head and neck and to the upper limbs. The Aorta passes down on the left of the spine to just below the second lumbar vertebra, where it divides into two great branches (Iliacs) which convey the blood to the organs in the pelvis and to the lower limbs.

ARTERIES OF THE HEAD AND NECK.

The Carotid Artery leaves the upper part of the chest and passes up on the side of the windpipe and, just below the level of the angle of the lower jaw, divides into the Internal and External Carotid Arteries. **The Internal Carotid Artery** ascends deeply in the neck, and enters the cranium to supply the brain with blood. **The External Carotid**

Artery gives off three important branches, the arteries of the tongue (Lingual), of the face (Facial) and of the back of the head (Occipital); the artery itself is then continued upwards to supply the scalp in the front half of the head (Temporal).

When a Carotid Artery is wounded, as in the case of a cut throat, apply the thumb of one hand on the artery at pressure point 1, pressing backwards against the spine (cervical vertebrae) and taking care to avoid the windpipe. (Fig. 60.) It may also be necessary to apply pressure with the other thumb above the wound to arrest the flow of blood (a) from the main vein in the neck (Jugular), which runs alongside the carotid artery and is usually wounded at the same time; (b) from the upper end of the carotid artery itself, which is often con-

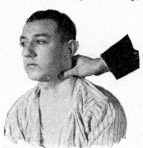

FIG. 60.
DIGITAL PRESSURE ON
CAROTID ARTERY.
(Pressure Point 1:)

siderable owing to communication between the branches of this artery and those of the corresponding one on the other side of the neck. Digital pressure must be maintained, by relays of assistants if necessary, until the doctor arrives.

The Facial Artery crosses the edge of the lower jaw in a slight hollow two fingers' breadth in front of the angle, and sends branches to the chin, lips, cheek, and outside of the nose. Hæmorrhage from wounds of the face below the level of the eye is to be arrested by :—

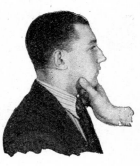

FIG. 61.

DIGITAL PRESSURE ON FACIAL ARTERY.

(Pressure Point 2.)

(*a*) Direct pressure on the wound from the outside of the cheek against the jaw bone.

(*b*) Grasping the wound of the lips or cheek by the finger inside and the thumb outside the mouth or vice versa.

(*c*) Indirect pressure on pressure point 2 (Fig. 61).

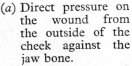

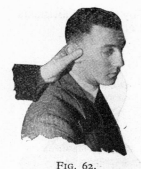

FIG. 62.
DIGITAL PRESSURE ON
TEMPORAL ARTERY.
(Pressure Point 3.)

The Temporal Artery may be felt pulsating in front of the upper part of the ear. Hæmorrhage from the region of the temple may be arrested by pressure applied on pressure point 3 (Fig. 62).

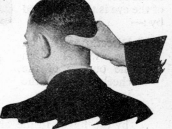

FIG. 63.
DIGITAL PRESSURE
ON OCCIPITAL
ARTERY.
(Pressure Point 4.)

The Occipital Artery supplies branches to the region of the scalp from behind the ear to the back of the head. Hæmorrhage from this region may be arrested by digital pressure on pressure point 4, four fingers' breadth behind the ear (Fig. 63). This point is difficult to find, and it is usually sufficient to apply pressure immediately below the wound.

Hæmorrhage from the Scalp may be arrested by applying a small firm pad on the bleeding point and securing it by a narrow bandage with its centre laid on the pad, the ends carried round the head in the direction most convenient, and tied tightly over the pad.

When a fracture is suspected in connection with a wound of the forehead or scalp, apply a ring pad around the seat of injury.

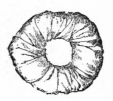

FIG. 64.

RING PAD.

RING PAD. To make a ring pad, pass one end of a narrow bandage round the fingers ; pass the other end of the bandage through the ring thus formed and continue to pass it through and through until the whole of the bandage is used and a ring as shown in Fig. 64 is formed.

ARTERIES OF THE UPPER LIMB.

The Subclavian Artery passes from a point behind the inner end of the collar-bone across the first rib to the armpit.

To apply digital pressure :—

  1.—Bare the neck and upper part of the chest.
  2.—Place the patient's arm against the body so as to depress the shoulder ; and cause him to incline his head towards the injured side.
  3.—Stand at the side of the patient opposite his shoulder, facing the patient.
  4.—Using the left hand for the right artery, and vice versa, grasp the neck low down, placing the fingers behind the shoulder and the thumb on pressure point 5 (Fig. 65) immediately above

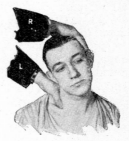

FIG. 65.
DIGITAL PRESSURE ON
SUBCLAVIAN ARTERY.
(Pressure Point 5.)

and behind the collar-bone in the hollow
between the muscles attached to the bone.

5.—Press the thumb deeply downwards
against the first rib, which is beneath the
collar-bone at this spot.

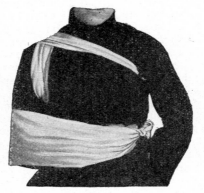

FIG. 66.
PRESSURE ON AXILLARY ARTERY BY PAD AND BANDAGE.
(Pressure Point 6.)

The Axillary Artery, which is a continuation of
the Subclavian, keeps close under the shoulder
joint, and can be felt pulsating when the fingers are

deeply pressed into the armpit. Digital pressure is difficult to apply to this artery.—

To apply a pad and bandage :—

    1.—Place a hard pad (the size of a billiard ball) in the armpit on pressure point 6.

    2.—Apply the centre of a narrow bandage on the pad ; cross the bandage on the shoulder, pull the ends tight and tie them under the opposite armpit, taking care that the pad does not slip.

    3.—Flex the forearm and tie the limb tightly to the trunk with a broad bandage, applied on a level with the elbow (Fig. 66).

The Brachial Artery is a continuation of the Axillary, and runs down the arm under the inner side of the biceps muscle, gradually passing forward until it reaches the middle of the front of the elbow. The inner seam of the coat-sleeve above the elbow roughly indicates its course.

To apply digital pressure on the Brachial artery (pressure point 7 Fig. 67) grasp the arm at its centre from behind (or from beneath if the arm is held as in Fig. 67) and compress the artery against the bone.

In an urgent emergency and if there is no possibility of a fracture, the Brachial artery may, as a purely temporary measure, be compressed at the elbow by flexion over a fold of the sleeve.

Just below the elbow the Brachial artery divides into the **Radial and Ulnar Arteries,** which run

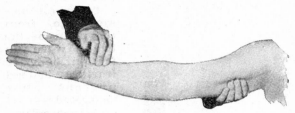

Fig. 67.

DIGITAL PRESSURE ON BRACHIAL ARTERY.
(Pressure Point 7.)
Note the taking of the pulse at the wrist.

along the front of the forearm on the outer and inner sides respectively. The pressure points (8 and 9) are about one inch above the wrist and about half an inch from the outer and inner sides of the forearm, where the arteries may be felt pulsating. These arteries join to form the **Palmar Arches** in the hand; branches run along on either side of each finger to the tip.

Pressure may be applied to the Radial and Ulnar arteries on pressure points 8 and 9, by the thumbs

(Fig. 68) or by means of two knots in a hand-kerchief tied tightly round the wrist.

To arrest hæmorrhage from the palm of the hand when a foreign body or fracture is not present nor suspected :—

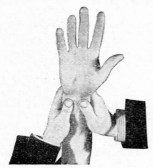

FIG. 68.
DIGITAL PRESSURE ON RADIAL
AND ULNAR ARTERIES.
(Pressure Points 8 and 9.)

1.—Apply a dressing and a firm pad, and make the patient grasp it.

2.—Spread out a triangular bandage, turn up the base about four inches, lay the back of the patient's hand on the centre of the bandage, fold the point over the knuckles and wrist, pass the two ends round the wrist, make the patient pull on the point of the bandage, cross the ends over the fingers and thumb twice and tie them as firmly as possible. Bring the point A down to

the knuckles and fasten with a safety pin
at B (Fig. 69).

3.—Apply a St. John sling.

Arterial hæmorrhage from the fingers may
be arrested by applying a small pad on the wound,
and securing it firmly with a bandage, strip of tape
or linen.

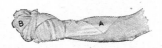

FIG. 69.
ARREST OF HÆMORRHAGE
FROM PALM BY PAD AND
BANDAGE.

ARTERIES OF THE LOWER LIMB.

The Femoral Artery, a continuation of the Iliac,
may be felt pulsating immediately below the skin
where it enters the thigh in the centre of the fold
of the groin. (To find the groin, raise the limb so as
to flex the thigh; the fold in the clothing at the top
of the thigh will indicate the groin.) The course
of the artery may be indicated by a line drawn from
the centre of the groin to the inner side of the knee.
After traversing two-thirds of this line, the Femoral

artery passes behind the thigh-bone to the back of the knee-joint as the **Popliteal artery.**

Digital pressure may be applied to the Femoral artery at the groin on pressure point 10 as follows :—

    1.—Lay the patient on his back.

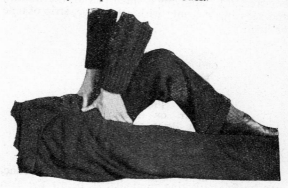

FIG. 70.
DIGITAL PRESSURE ON FEMORAL ARTERY.
(Pressure Point 10.)

    2.—Kneel beside the patient, facing his head.

    3.—Place the thumbs one on the other upon the pressure point, at the centre of the groin, grasping the thigh with the hands (Fig. 70).

    4.—Press firmly against the brim of the pelvis.

When the Femoral artery is wounded in the upper third of its course, pressure must be maintained at the groin. No really satisfactory tourniquet has been devised for compression at this point, and relays of assistants should be employed to keep up the pressure until the doctor arrives ; each fresh assistant places his thumbs over those of his predecessor, who slips his away, and thus gushes of blood are prevented during the change.

Application of a tourniquet to the Femoral artery (pressure point II) :—

When practising compression of this artery, it is a good plan to draw a chalk line from the centre of the groin to the inner side of the knee and place the pad of the tourniquet on this line as high up as the bandage can be applied. The pad should be the size of a lawn tennis ball.

Just below and behind the knee-joint the Popliteal artery divides into the **Anterior** (front) and **Posterior** (back) **Tibial arteries.**

The Posterior Tibial Artery passes down the back of the leg to the inner side of the ankle. It is at first deeply placed between the muscles of the calf, but it approaches the surface as it proceeds, so that it can be felt pulsating midway between the inner ankle and heel. As it enters the sole it divides into the **Plantar Arteries,** which run forward amongst the muscles to supply the foot.

The Anterior Tibial Artery, on leaving the Popliteal, at once passes forward between the leg bones, and, deeply placed amongst the muscles, runs down the leg to the centre of the front of the ankle. This artery is continued as the **Dorsal Artery of the Foot,** which, passing forward over the tarsus, dips down to the sole between the first and second metatarsal bones. This artery joins with the Plantar arteries to form the **Plantar Arch,** from which branches run along on either side of each toe to the tip.

At the ankle, pressure may be applied by the fingers or by pads and a bandage on pressure points 12 and 13.

To arrest hæmorrhage from the sole of the foot when a foreign body or fracture is not present nor suspected :—

    1.—Apply a dressing and a firm pad over the bleeding point.

    2.—Maintain firm pressure by placing the centre of a narrow bandage over the pad, cross the bandage over the instep, carry the two ends round the ankle, cross them again over the instep and tie tightly over the pad.

    3.—Support the foot in an elevated position.

General Rules for Treatment of a Wound accompanied by Capillary Hæmorrhage.

1.—Expose the wound, removing whatever clothing may be necessary.

2.—Remove any foreign bodies, such as broken glass, bits of clothing, hair, which can be seen lying loose in the wound ; do not search for foreign bodies which cannot be seen.

3.—If the wound is obviously dirty, and medical aid cannot be procured, wash away as much of the dirt as possible by gently pouring sterilised water over it freely, notwithstanding the fact that wounds heal best if kept dry. **Never wash the surrounding parts towards a wound.**

4.—Apply an antiseptic all over the wound and the surrounding skin, and cover with a dry dressing.

5.—Cover the dressing with cotton wool, lint or other soft material.

6.—Apply a bandage over the dressing firmly ; but if the presence of a foreign body or fracture is suspected, apply it lightly.

GENERAL RULES FOR TREATMENT OF A WOUND
ACCOMPANIED BY VENOUS HÆMORRHAGE.

1.—Place the patient in a suitable position, bearing in mind that blood escapes with less force when the patient sits, and still less when he lies down.

2.—Elevate the bleeding part, except in the case of a fractured limb.

3.—Expose the wound, removing whatever clothing may be necessary.

4.—Apply direct digital pressure, except over a fracture or foreign body.

5.—Remove any constrictions, such as collar or garters, from the heart side of the wound.

6.—Apply a firm bandage round the limb near the wound on the side away from the heart.

7.—Remove any foreign bodies, such as broken glass, bits of clothing, hair, which can be seen lying loose in the wound ; do not search for foreign bodies which cannot be seen.

8.—If the wound is obviously dirty, and medical aid cannot be procured, wash away as much of the dirt as possible by gently pouring sterilised water over it freely notwithstanding the fact that wounds heal best if kept dry. **Never wash the surrounding parts towards a wound.**

9.—Apply an antiseptic all over the wound and the surrounding skin, and cover with a dry dressing.

10.—Cover the dressing with cotton wool, lint or other soft material.

11.—Apply a bandage over the dressing firmly ; but if the presence of a foreign body or fracture is suspected apply it lightly.

12.—Support the injured part.

Hæmorrhage from a Varicose Vein.

A varicose vein is a permanently dilated or over-stretched vein whose walls have lost their elasticity, and has bead-like projections along its course. The veins of the leg are specially apt to become varicose from several causes, such as long standing or tight garters. The first effect is to throw extra work upon the valves, and the bead-like projections are caused by the blood accumulating in the pockets behind the valves. In time the vein becomes so dilated that the valves can no longer span it, thus allowing the backward flow of blood, so that in bleeding from a ruptured varicose vein the blood may flow from both sides of the wound.

Treatment.

1.—Lay the patient down, and, except in the case of a fracture, raise the leg at a right angle to the body.

E

2.—Expose the wound.

3.—Apply direct digital pressure.

4.—Remove any constriction from the limb.

5.—Apply a bandage firmly on the side of the wound furthest from the heart.

6.—Apply a second bandage between the wound and the heart.

7.—Apply an antiseptic all over the wound and the surrounding skin, and cover with a dry dressing.

8.—Cover the dressing with cotton wool, lint or other soft material.

9.—Apply a bandage over the dressing firmly; but if the presence of a foreign body or fracture is suspected apply it lightly.

10.—Keep the leg elevated.

WOUND OF THE ABDOMINAL WALL.

TREATMENT.

A. When there is no protrusion of organs :—

1(*a*).—If the wound is vertical, keep the patient flat on his back with the lower limbs straight.

(*b*).—If the wound is transverse, keep the patient on his back, draw the knees well up and raise the head and shoulders.

2.—Apply an antiseptic, and a dry dressing to the wound.

3.—Fix the dressing in position with a broad bandage tied tightly.

4.—Keep the patient warm.

5.—Give nothing by the mouth.

B. When internal organs such as the intestines protrude through the wound, whether vertical or transverse :—

1.—Keep the patient on his back, draw the knees well up and raise the head and shou'ders.

2.—Make no attempt to replace organs, but cover them with lint or a soft towel wrung out of sterilised hot water (at the temperature of the body 98.4°) to which may be added, if readily available, salt in the proportion of one teaspoonful to a pint of water. Change the application every fifteen minutes.

3.—Cover the application with cotton wool or soft clean flannel.

4.—Apply hot water bottles to both sides of the body ; and keep the patient warm, avoiding undue pressure on the abdomen.

5.—Give nothing by the mouth.

6.—Remove the patient to hospital **as speedily as possible.**

WOUNDS CAUSED BY A VENOMOUS SNAKE OR RABID ANIMAL.

SNAKE BITE.

The bite of a venomous snake endangers life and immediate action is necessary to prevent the spread of the venom throughout the body.

TREATMENT.

A. If the bite is on a limb—

1.—**Immediately** arrest circulation in the limb by means of a **constriction** on the upper arm or thigh (as the case may be) between the wound and the heart. It is useless to place the constriction round the forearm or leg.

The constriction may consist of rubber tubing or elastic braces ; or strips of clothing, a tie, handkerchief or non-elastic braces, placed loosely round the limb and tightened with a stick (as in an improvised tourniquet). The constriction should be kept in position for twenty minutes, then relaxed for one minute or until the skin becomes pink, and again tightened. Repeat this procedure until the arrival of a doctor.

2.—Keep the patient absolutely at rest.

3.—If the patient is able to swallow give hot drinks such as strong coffee, tea or milk. Alcohol should be avoided.

4.—As the natural alarm of the patient will seriously aggravate the condition it is of the utmost importance to reassure him with encouraging words.

5.—Wash the wound, preferably with a weak (pale pink) solution of permanganate of potash, in order to remove any venom which may have dried on the skin.

6.—If breathing is failing apply artificial respiration (see page 144).

B. If the bite is elsewhere than on a limb— adopt rules 2, 3, 4, 5 and 6 pending the arrival of a doctor.

BITE BY A RABID ANIMAL—HYDROPHOBIA.

Hydrophobia is caused by the bite of an animal such as a dog, jackal, fox or wolf suffering from rabies. The virus travels from the bite along the nerves to the central nervous system, and differs entirely in this respect from snake bite where the venom is absorbed directly into the veins from the bitten tissues.

TREATMENT.

1.—After a person has been bitten by a rabid animal or one suspected of having rabies, every effort should be made to promote bleeding so as to wash the wound from within outwards.   This is best done by :—

(a) **Immediately** placing a **constriction** (a piece of cord, tape or handkerchief) between the bite and the trunk tightly enough to cause congestion of the limb and ensure bleeding, but not so tightly as to obstruct the arterial circulation in which case the limb becomes pallid, the pulse cannot be felt and bleeding entirely ceases.

(b) Keeping the affected part low : the upper limb should be allowed to hang down and in the case of the lower limb the patient should be seated with the foot on the ground.

(c) Bathing the wound with warm water to which crystals of permanganate of potash have been added : the solution should be pale pink in colour.

2.—Give alcohol such as brandy or whisky (in the case of an adult two tablespoonfuls or in the case of a child two teaspoonfuls in a wine-glass of water) or hot black coffee.

3.—If it is not possible to obtain the services of a doctor **within a few minutes** of the person being bitten, the wound should be cauterised.   This is best done by removing the constriction and applying a fluid caustic, such as carbolic or nitric acid on a match or a piece of wood cut to a point, or lunar caustic. To prove effective every tooth mark must be probed and cauterised separately, as only by so doing can the virus be destroyed.

If more than half an hour has elapsed since the person has been bitten, proceed as in rules 1 and 2 and then remove the constriction, but do not cauterise the wound.

4.—Apply a dry dressing and retain it in position with a bandage.

CHAPTER X.

HÆMORRHAGE FROM SPECIAL REGIONS.

HÆMORRHAGE FROM AN INTERNAL ORGAN.

Hæmorrhage from an internal organ may be caused by injury, such as a crush, blow, fracture of a rib or pelvis, or by a stab or bullet, or may be due to disease, in which case no external cause is apparent.

The signs and symptoms are :—

1.—Pallor of the face and lips, and cold clammy skin.

2.—Rapid loss of strength, giddiness and faintness, especially when the upright position is assumed.

3.—Breathing hurried and laboured, and accompanied by yawning and sighing.

4.—The pulse fails, and may altogether disappear at the wrist.

5.—The patient throws his arms about, tugs at the clothing round the neck, and calls for air (air hunger).

6.—Finally the patient may become totally unconscious.

In **Hæmorrhage from the Lungs** the blood will be coughed up bright red and frothy.

In **Hæmorrhage from the Stomach** the blood is vomited and sometimes has the appearance of coffee grounds.

In **Hæmorrhage from the Liver, Spleen, Pancreas or Intestines,** the bleeding is accompanied by pain and swelling at the seat of injury.

In **Hæmorrhage from the Kidneys** blood will escape with the urine, and there may be pain and swelling over the injured kidney.

In **Hæmorrhage from the Bladder** the signs and symptoms are either inability to pass water, or, if a little is passed, it is tinged with blood. The bladder may be injured by a fracture of the pelvis.

TREATMENT.

1.—Remove the patient to hospital as soon as possible, taking special care to lessen the effects of shock.

2.—If the seat of the hæmorrhage is known, apply an ice bag or a cold compress over the region.

3.—Give nothing by the mouth except in hæmorrhage from the lungs, when ice may be given to suck

E*

HÆMORRHAGE FROM THE CHEEK, THE TONGUE, THE GUMS, THE SOCKET OF A TOOTH, OR THE THROAT.

TREATMENT.

Give ice or cold water to hold in the mouth.

If bleeding from the front part of the cheek or the tongue is excessive, compress the part by a piece of clean lint held between the finger and thumb.

If the bleeding is from the socket of a tooth, plug the socket with a piece of clean lint or cotton wool ; over this place a small cork or other substance of suitable size, and instruct the patient to bite on it.

This hæmorrhage must not be confused with hæmorrhage from the lungs or stomach.

HÆMORRHAGE FROM THE NOSE.

TREATMENT.

1.—Place the patient in a sitting position in a current of air before an open window, with the head thrown slightly back and the hands raised above the head.

2.—Undo all tight clothing around the neck and chest.

3.—Cause the patient to keep the mouth open, and so avoid breathing through the nose.

4.—Apply cold over the nose and also the spine at the level of the collar ; place the feet in hot water.

5.—Warn the patient not to blow the nose.

HÆMORRHAGE FROM THE EAR CHANNEL.

Blood issuing from the Ear Channel generally indicates a fracture of the base of the skull.

TREATMENT.

1.—Make no attempt to plug the ear.

2.—Apply a dry dressing over the ear and bandage lightly.

BRUISES.

A blow anywhere on the surface of the body may cause extensive capillary hæmorrhage beneath the skin, without breaking it—a " black eye " is an instance. The injury is accompanied by discoloration and swelling.

TREATMENT.

Apply pieces of lint soaked in equal parts of spirit and water, or a cold compress.

Chapter XI.

THE RESPIRATORY SYSTEM.

The organs concerned in Respiration are the Nose, the Throat, the Windpipe (Trachea), the Air Tubes (Bronchi) and Air Cells (Lungs).

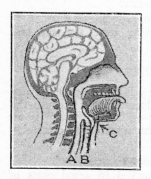 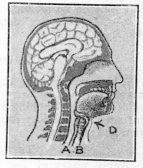

Fig. 71.   Fig. 72.

VERTICAL SECTION OF HEAD.

A. GULLET.   B. WINDPIPE.

C. EPIGLOTTIS OPEN.   D. EPIGLOTTIS CLOSED.

Air is conveyed by the nostrils (or mouth) to the back of the throat, whence it enters the windpipe by an opening guarded by a flap (the epiglottis) against the entry of solids or fluids. During insensibility however, the flap may fail to act, so that, should solids or fluids be given by the mouth, they may enter the windpipe and cause choking. Another danger is that the tongue of an insensible person is very apt to fall back on the flap, and so obstruct the windpipe. (Figs. 71 and 72.) The windpipe extends to two inches below the top of the breast-bone, where it divides into the right and left bronchus. Each bronchus enters a lung and divides into small and still smaller bronchial tubes, until the ultimate recesses of the lung—the air cells or air spaces—are reached.

The **Lungs,** Right and Left, occupy the greater part of the chest, and lie immediately within the ribs. Each lung is enveloped in a fine membrane (the pleura), which allows it to move within the chest freely during breathing.

Respiration, or breathing, consists of two acts— Inspiration, an enlargement of the chest cavity, during which air is drawn into the lungs, and Expiration, a diminution of the chest, during which air is driven out of the lungs. A pause follows the act of expiration. In health fifteen to eighteen

Insensible patient
— no fluid

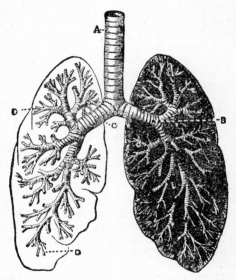

FIG. 73.—THE LUNGS AND BRONCHIAL TUBES.
A. Trachea, or Windpipe. B. Left Bronchus. C. Right
Bronchus. D. Smaller Bronchial Tubes.

breaths are taken per minute, and at each inspiration about twenty to thirty cubic inches of air enter the lungs, and a similar quantity is expelled at each expiration.

The enlargement and diminution of the chest cavity are effected partly by the muscles of respiration attached to the ribs, but chiefly by the diaphragm, the large arched muscular partition which separates the chest from the abdomen. In inspiration, which is a muscular act, the ribs are raised, and the diaphragm contracts and becomes flattened, thus increasing the capacity of the chest, tending to produce a vacuum and causing air to enter. In expiration, an act performed without muscular effort, the ribs fall and the arch of the diaphragm rises; this lessens the capacity of the chest and forces air out. In the capillaries of the lungs the air gives off to the blood its oxygen and takes up from it carbonic acid gas, heat and water; thus the air expired becomes warmer and contains carbonic acid and watery vapour, and the impure dark red blood becomes purified and of a bright red colour.

As the blood depends upon air for its purification and the oxygen necessary to maintain life, interference with breathing very soon may produce a dangerous state called **asphyxia**, examples of which are afforded by drowning, suffocation, choking, etc.

It should not, however, be assumed that the patient is dead because breathing is not apparent. Prompt steps should be taken to **ensure that breathing is possible,** i.e., that the air passages are not obstructed, that pressure does not prevent the necessary expansion of the chest and that there is an abundance of pure air.

If natural breathing is seen to be failing or cannot be discerned, artificial means of restoring it must be resorted to at once as follows :—

ARTIFICIAL RESPIRATION.

SCHAFER'S METHOD.

1.—**Adjust the patient's position.**—At once lay the patient in a prone position (i.e., back upwards), with arms extended above the head, and his head turned to one side, so as to keep his nose and mouth away from the ground (Fig. 74). Do not waste time by loosening clothing ; no pad is to be placed under the patient, nor need the tongue be drawn out, as it will fall naturally towards the lips.

To turn the patient to the prone position, stoop at his side, place his arms close to the body, cross his far leg over his near leg, and, protecting his face with one hand, with the other grasp the clothing at the hip on the opposite side of the body and pull smartly over.

2.—Imitate the movements of breathing.

(a) *Induce expiration.*—Kneel at one side of the patient, facing his head and sitting on your heels

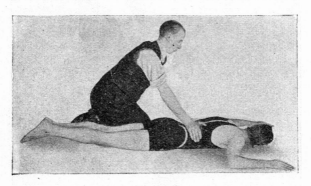

FIG. 74.
ARTIFICIAL RESPIRATION.
(Schafer's Method.)

(Fig. 74). Place your hands on the small of the patient's back, their lower edges just clearing the top of the pelvis, the wrists nearly touching, the thumbs as near each other as possible without strain and the fingers passing over the loins on either side and pointing towards the ground but not spread out (Fig. 75). Bending your body from

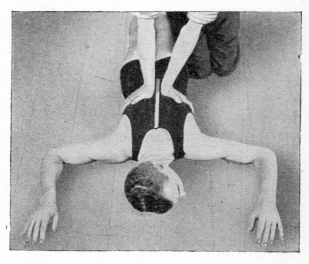

FIG. 75.
ARTIFICIAL RESPIRATION.
(Schafer's Method.)

the knees and somewhat straightening the hip-joints swing slowly forward keeping your arms quite straight and rigid so that the weight of your body is conveyed to your hands directly downwards

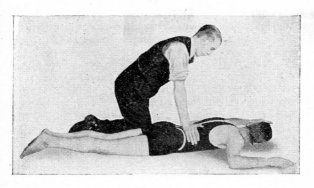

FIG. 76.
ARTIFICIAL RESPIRATION.
(Schafer's Method.)

(Fig. 76). No exertion is required ; the necessary pressure is imparted by the weight of your body. In this way the patient's abdomen is pressed against the ground ; the abdominal organs are forced against the diaphragm ; the diaphragm rises and air is driven out of the lungs together with any water or mucus which may be present in the air passages or in the mouth, producing **Expiration.**

(*b*) *Induce inspiration.*—Swing your body slowly backwards to its first position thus removing the weight from the hands (which are kept in position) and relaxing the pressure on the abdomen (Fig. 74).

The organs now assume their former position, the diaphragm descends, the thorax is enlarged and air passes into the lungs, producing **Inspiration.**

(*c*) *Alternate these movements* by a rhythmic swaying forwards and backwards of your body from the knee joints, twelve times a minute. The rhythm is—pressure two seconds and relaxation three seconds.

When natural breathing begins, regulate the movements of artificial respiration to correspond with it, and promote circulation by rubbing the limbs vigorously towards the heart and by applying warmth.

Watch the patient carefully for some time to see that the breathing does not fail ; if it does, at once resort again to artificial respiration.

Artificial respiration must be continued perseveringly until respiration is restored or until a doctor pronounces life to be extinct.

SILVESTER'S METHOD.

This method is to be used only when it is impossible to turn the patient on to his face.

1.—Adjust the patient's position.—Without wasting a moment, place the patient on his back on a flat surface, inclined if possible from the feet upwards. Undo all tight clothing. Raise and support the shoulders on a small, firm cushion or folded article of dress placed under the shoulder-blades.

2.—Maintain a free entrance of air into the windpipe.—An assistant must catch hold of the patient's tongue with a handkerchief, draw it forward as far as possible, and hold it in that position. If this is not done there is great danger of obstruction of the windpipe by the tongue falling back over the top of it (compare Figs. 71 and 72, p. 140).

3.—Imitate the movements of breathing.

(a) *Induce inspiration.*—Kneel at a convenient distance behind the patient's head, and, grasping his forearms just below the elbows, draw the arms upwards, outwards, and towards you, with a sweeping movement, making the elbows touch the ground

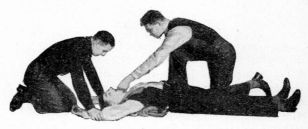

FIG. 77.
ARTIFICIAL RESPIRATION.
(Silvester's Method.)

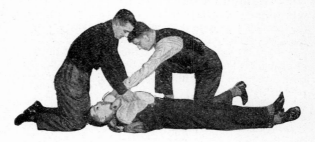

FIG. 78.
ARTIFICIAL RESPIRATION.
(Silvester's Method.)

(Fig. 77). The cavity of the chest is thus enlarged, and air is drawn into the lungs.

(b) *Induce expiration.*—Bring the patient's flexed arms slowly forwards, downwards and inwards, press the arms and elbows firmly on the chest on each side of the breast-bone (Fig. 78). By this means air is expelled from the lungs.

(c) *Repeat* these movements alternately, deliberately, and perseveringly about twelve times a minute. The rhythm is—pressure two seconds and relaxation three seconds.

When natural breathing begins, regulate the movements of artificial respiration to correspond with it, and promote circulation by rubbing the limbs vigorously towards the heart and by applying warmth.

Watch the patient carefully for some time to see that the breathing does not fail; if it does, at once resort again to artificial respiration.

Artificial respiration must be continued perseveringly until respiration is restored or until a doctor pronounces life to be extinct.

Chapter XII.

THE NERVOUS SYSTEM.

Two systems of nerves, the Cerebro-spinal and the Sympathetic, regulate and control the movements and functions of the body.

The Cerebro-spinal System.

The Cerebro-spinal System is made up of the Brain, Spinal Cord and Nerves ; through its agency sensations are received and the will causes the action of the voluntary muscles. For example, when a part is injured a sensation of pain is conveyed to the brain by the sensory fibres of the nerve, thus affording an indication of the seat of injury, or a warning of a possible danger of further damage. On attention being directed to the injury, motor fibres of the nerve convey a message to the muscles, and an attempt is instantly made to ease the pain by moving the injured part.

The **Brain,** situated within the cranium, is the seat of intellect, the emotions, and the will ; it is the organ where impressions brought by sensory nerves are received, and from which orders are given through the motor nerves.

The **Spinal Cord,** coming from the brain, consists of nerve tissue and lies within the spinal canal. · It leaves the brain through an opening in the base of the skull, and extends to the second lumbar vertebra.

The **Nerves** proceed from the brain and spinal cord in pairs as pearly-white trunks, and their branches can be traced throughout the tissues of the body. When a nerve is severed there is loss of power and sensation in the region in which its branches are distributed.

THE SYMPATHETIC SYSTEM.

The Sympathetic System consists of a network of bodies of nerve tissue (ganglia) and connecting nerves ; it controls the involuntary muscles, and regulates the vital functions of the body. The main part of the network (solar plexus) is situated in the upper part of the abdomen behind the stomach ; when it is struck, as in " winding " in football and boxing, severe collapse may result. The Sympathetic System is not under the control of the will, and acts alike during sleep and activity.

A — apoplexy
I — intoxication
D — disease —
epilepsy

CHAPTER XIII.

INSENSIBILITY.

Insensibility is loss of consciousness due to interruption of the action of the brain brought about by some interference with the functions of the nervous system. Apart from natural sleep there are two degrees of insensibility which may be partial (Stupor) or complete (Coma).

In stupor the patient can be aroused with some difficulty, but not at all in coma. In stupor the pupils of the eyes (the black part surrounded by the coloured iris) respond to light—that is, contract in a bright light and expand or dilate when the light is shaded, but not in coma. Also the patient will object to the eyeballs being touched in the former but not in the latter state.

GENERAL RULES FOR TREATMENT OF INSENSIBILITY.

1.—If breathing is absent perform artificial respiration.

2.—If breathing is present lay the patient on his back with his head turned on one side and

> (a) If the face is pale, keep the head and shoulders low and raise the feet.

F — faint
I — injury — head
R — respiration
S — shock
T — terminal unconscious

    (*b*) If the face is flushed, raise the head and shoulders.

3.—Undo all clothing about the neck, chest and waist.

4.—Ensure an abundance of fresh air. Open windows and doors ; keep back a crowd ; remove from harmful gases or impure atmosphere.

5.—Adopt the special treatment appropriate for the condition which has caused the insensibility.

6.—Remove the patient to shelter in a recumbent position as soon as expedient.

7.—Give no food or fluids whatever by the mouth while the patient is insensible.

8.—Unless unavoidable, never leave the patient until he has been placed in the charge of another responsible person.

9.—On return to consciousness water may be given to drink in sips. If the pulse is feeble give hot, strong tea or coffee, provided hæmorrhage, either external or from an internal organ, is not apparent or suspected. A desire to sleep should be encouraged, except in cases of hypnotic poisoning, a condition that may generally be recognised by the history of the case, and also by the pupils of the eyes being minutely contracted (pin-point pupils).

A. INSENSIBILITY WHEN BREATHING IS ABSENT (ASPHYXIA).

A continuous want of pure air produces a condition known as **Asphyxia**, which will cause loss of consciousness (**Insensibility**). Asphyxia may be brought about as follows :—

I. Obstruction of the air passages.

(a) BY DROWNING.

(b) BY PRESSURE FROM OUTSIDE : Strangulation, hanging, smothering.

(c) BY A FOREIGN BODY (e.g., a piece of food, false teeth, etc.) IN THE THROAT : Choking.

(d) BY SWELLING OF THE TISSUES OF THE THROAT : Inflammation, scald of the throat, poisoning by a corrosive, or stings of insects.

II. Inhaling poisonous gases, such as coal gas (as used in the house), water gas, smoke, fumes from a charcoal or coke fire or motor exhaust, sewer gas, lime-kiln gas.

III. Pressure on the chest, as when crushed by sand or debris, or by a crowd.

IV. Nervous affections, as the result of certain poisons (see Chapter XIV), electric shock, or stroke by lightning.

convulsion.
gag

flat back
face side
keep warm

Treatment of Asphyxia.

1.—Remove the cause of the asphyxia or the patient from the cause—whichever is more expedient.

2.—Adopt the general rules for the treatment of insensibility as far as applicable.

Additional Treatment in Special Cases.

Drowning.

While artificial respiration is being performed instruct bystanders to remove wet clothing as far as possible, and to wrap the patient in dry blankets or other clothing.

Strangulation.

Cut and remove the band constricting the throat.

Hanging.

Do not wait for a policeman : grasp the lower limbs and raise the body to take the tension off the rope ; cut the rope, and free the neck.

Choking.

To dislodge the obstruction bend the head and shoulders forward and thump the back hard between the shoulder-blades. If this is unsuccessful encourage vomiting by passing two fingers right to the back of the throat.

Swelling of the tissues of the Throat.

If possible, place the patient before the fire. Apply a hot compress to the front of the neck, from the chin to the top of the breast-bone ; renew the hot compress frequently. If breathing has not ceased or has been restored, give ice to suck or, failing ice, cold water to drink ; butter, olive or salad oil or medicinal paraffin may also be given (see page 172).

Suffocation by Smoke.

Before entering a building or room full of smoke tie a handkerchief, wet if possible, over the nose and mouth. Keep low, and quickly but cautiously drag the patient out.

Suffocation by Poisonous Gas.

On entering any enclosed space known or suspected to contain poisonous gas of any kind ensure a free circulation of air by opening or breaking doors and windows.

Hold your breath, keep low and remove the patient as quickly as possible.

In cases where ventilation is not possible and the character of the gas is known to be deadly a suitable gas mask should be worn.

ELECTRIC SHOCK.

If it is impossible to switch off the current immediately, precautions must be taken to prevent the person rendering assistance from receiving a dangerous, or even fatal shock. He should therefore protect himself by standing, if possible, on a dry non-conducting material which will resist the current, such as india-rubber, linoleum, glass or any other non-metallic substance. He should similarly protect his hands with india-rubber gloves, tobacco pouch, mackintosh or other article of dry clothing.

If no means of protection are at hand, an attempt may be made to drag the patient away by means of a loop of dry rope or a crooked stick ; an umbrella is not safe because the metal ribs would act as conductors of electricity, and it is not infrequently the case that the " stick " of the umbrella is a metal tube. Care should be taken to avoid touching with naked hands the patient's skin, wet clothing, or boots if the soles are nailed. The armpits should be avoided, as perspiration usually makes the clothing damp there.

In electric shock the act of breathing is suspended and efforts at natural breathing will be renewed only if artificial respiration is **started at**

once and effectively performed for a long time.
Shock is severe and burns are frequently present.

The patient must be cautioned not to resume physical or mental activity without the consent of a doctor however slight the shock may have been.

B. (1) INSENSIBILITY WHEN BREATHING IS PRESENT AND THERE ARE CONVULSIONS.

Convulsions are spasmodic and involuntary contractions of the muscles of the body and limbs; they may be general or they may be limited to the limbs on one side of the body.

1.—CONSTITUTIONAL CAUSES.

(a) **Epilepsy** is a sudden and complete loss of consciousness in persons of any age, but usually in young adults.

The signs usually present are—the patient falls to the ground, sometimes with a scream, and passes into a state of convulsion affecting the whole of the body and limbs, which may in consequence be injured through contact with surrounding objects; the face is flushed at first and rapidly becomes livid; frothing at the mouth and biting of the tongue may occur.

SPECIAL TREATMENT.

1.—Pull the patient away from a source of danger, such as machinery, a wall or fireplace, to prevent him hurting himself. Light pieces of furniture should be moved out of the way.

2.—Support the patient's head, and after wrapping a pencil or similar hard substance in a handkerchief, hold it between his back teeth to prevent the tongue being bitten. Do not forcibly restrain the patient's movements.

3.—Adopt the general rules for treatment of Insensibility as far as applicable.

(b) **In Hysterical Fits (Hysteria)** the patient, often a young girl, suddenly loses command of her feelings and actions, in consequence of mental excitement. She subsides on a couch or in some comfortable position, throws herself about, grinding her teeth and clenching her fists ; she clutches at anyone or anything near her, kicks, cries and laughs alternately. The eyeballs may be turned upwards, and the eyelids opened and shut rapidly. At times froth appears at the lips, and other irregular symptoms may develop. Complete insensibility is not present.

SPECIAL TREATMENT.

Avoid sympathy with the patient, speak firmly to her and leave her by herself.

(c) **Infantile Convulsions.**

The signs usually present are—twitching of the muscles of the limbs and trunk ; extreme pallor and later blueness of the face ; occasional squinting ; " holding of the breath " and froth at the mouth.

SPECIAL TREATMENT.

1.—Strip the child and support it in a hot bath so that the water covers the whole of the body up to the neck and keep it there until the convulsions have ceased or the doctor arrives. Keep a sponge frequently dipped in cold water on the top of the head as long as the child is in the bath.

2.—On removal from the bath, wrap the child in a warm blanket but still keep the head cool.

3.—If the convulsions recur repeat the treatment.

4.—Adopt as far as applicable the general rules for treatment of Insensibility.

2.—POISONING.

(a) Prussic Acid and Cyanide of Potassium.
(b) Fungi and berries, in the later stages.

For signs, symptoms and treatment, see Poisons (Chapter XIV.).

B. (2) INSENSIBILITY WHEN BREATHING IS PRESENT AND THERE ARE *NO* CONVULSIONS.

(1) INJURIES TO THE HEAD.

(*a*) **Concussion of the brain (stunning) is a** disturbance of the functions of the brain caused by a blow or fall on the head, or by a fall on the feet or lower part of the spine.

The signs are :—The patient is at once in a state of stupor, which may last for a short time only, or may deepen into coma. The face is pale, the pulse quick and weak, the breathing shallow and the skin cold.

(*b*) **Compression of the brain** may result from the same causes as produce Concussion ; in fact Compression is frequently preceded by Concussion. Signs of injury are usually present, and the condition is due to pressure on the brain by a blood clot or piece of bone in fracture of the skull.

The signs are :—The face is flushed ; the pulse full and slow ; the breathing becomes stertorous ; loss of power and sensation may be only partial and not complete ; there may be discharge of blood from the nose and ear (fractured base of skull); the pupil of one eye may be larger than that of the other, and the temperature of the body raised.

Compression of the brain differs from Concussion also in the fact that the signs may not appear at once, but may be delayed for a time.

SPECIAL TREATMENT OF INJURIES TO THE HEAD.

1.—Adopt the general rules for treatment of Insensibility as far as applicable.

2.—Promote warmth in the lower part of the body by applying hot water bottles to the sides of the abdomen and lower limbs.

3.—Apply ice or cold water to the head continuously. Merely sprinkling the head with cold water acts as a stimulant to the circulation in the head, and does more harm than good.

4.—Keep the patient absolutely quiet in a darkened room.

No case of head injury should be regarded lightly, and a caution should be given to a patient who has been unconscious, even for only a moment, not to resume physical or mental activity without the consent of a doctor.

(2) OTHER CAUSES.

(*a*) **Shock and Collapse**.

(*b*) **Fainting** (syncope) is a condition due to sudden failure of the action of the heart, which may be caused by hæmorrhage; or by fatigue, want of food, or a close or crowded room; or by fright, dread, sudden bad news, or by the sudden relief from fear or anxiety after prolonged suspense.

The signs are:—The patient turns giddy and falls; the face is pale; the pulse is rapid and weak, or almost imperceptible; the breathing is quick, sighing and irregular, and the skin becomes cold and clammy.

SPECIAL TREATMENT.

1.—Adopt the general rules for treatment of Insensibility as far as applicable.

2.—Sprinkle the face with hot and cold water alternately, and apply warmth to the pit of the stomach and over the heart; vigorous friction of the limbs upwards has a stimulating effect. Smelling salts may be held to the nose.

3.—If bleeding has been the cause of the condition guard against its recurrence. The wound will not bleed to any marked extent while the action of the heart is feeble. The wound must be carefully watched to be sure that bleeding does not recur when the patient begins to regain consciousness and the heart's action improves; or, if there is no wound, look for signs of hæmorrhage from an internal organ.

If want of nourishment has been the cause of the condition give food sparingly at first.

(c) **Apoplexy** (a " stroke ") usually occurs in elderly people, and is due to the rupture of a diseased blood vessel causing hæmorrhage into the brain tissue ; signs of injury are not necessarily present.

The signs usually present are :—the face is flushed ; the pulse full and slow ; the breathing stertorous ; one side of the body more limp than the other, and the pupil of one eye larger than that of the other ; the temperature of the body raised.

SPECIAL TREATMENT.

1.—Adopt the general rules for treatment of Insensibility as far as applicable.

2.—Promote warmth in the lower part of the body by applying hot water bottles to the lower limbs and feet.

3.—Apply ice or cold water to the head continuously.

(d) **Sunstroke or Heatstroke** may be caused by exposure to the rays of the sun during a march in very hot weather when heavily burdened, or to great heat, as in the stoke-hole of a steamer, especially in the tropics.

The signs and symptoms are—the face is very flushed; the pulse quick and bounding; the breathing is difficult; the patient develops sickness, faintness, giddiness, thirst; the skin becomes dry and burning. A very high temperature, stertorous breathing and insensibility (either stupor or coma) may ensue.

In Sunstroke or Heatstroke congestion extends not only to the brain but to the whole of the spinal cord; consequently the area to be relieved is greater than that in apoplexy, and different treatment is necessary.

SPECIAL TREATMENT.

1.—Adopt the general rules for treatment of Insensibility as far as applicable.

2.—Remove the patient to a cool, shady spot, and strip him to the waist.

3.—Sponge the body with cold water continuously, and apply ice bags to the head and spine until the symptoms subside.

4.—Fan him vigorously.

5.—When consciousness returns give Epsom or Glauber Salts, a tablespoonful to a tumbler of water.

6.—Give drinks of cold water freely.

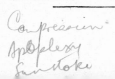

Compression
Apoplexy
Sunstroke

Chapter XIV.

POISONS.

A poison is any substance which when taken into the body in sufficient quantity is capable of destroying life.

It may be taken either accidentally or intentionally:—

(a) By the mouth.

(b) Through the lungs, by the inhalation of poisonous gases or fumes. (Asphyxia.)

(c) By injection under the skin.

Poisons may be divided into two classes:—

1. THOSE WHICH BURN THE LIPS AND MOUTH.
   Corrosives, which actually burn parts with which they come in contact, and thus cause intense pain, corrosion of mouth and throat, and possibly retching, difficulty in breathing and collapse.
   These consist of the strong acids and alkalies.

2. THOSE WHICH DO NOT BURN THE LIPS AND MOUTH.

(a) **Irritants,** which do not burn but when taken by the mouth cause an irritating sensation in throat and stomach and retching, generally accompanied by colic and diarrhœa.

These include metallic poisons, poisonous fungi and berries and decomposing food. When several persons, who have partaken of the same food, develop similar signs and symptoms, such as vomiting, colicky pains and diarrhœa, ptomaine poisoning due to decomposing food should be suspected.

(b) **Hypnotics,** which at once induce a tendency to go to sleep, developing into stupor and later coma. These include opium and its preparations, in which the pupils become minutely contracted—pin-point pupils. They also include those tablets and preparations which are used to relieve pain and induce sleep. In both groups the breathing becomes deep and stertorous, the pulse slow and weak, the face livid and the skin cold and clammy.

F*

(c) **Deliriants,** those which produce at first delirium, developing later into coma. The pupils are dilated and the pulse quick. These include belladonna, stramonium, chloroform and alcohol.

(d) **Convulsants,** which produce convulsions. There is a feeling of suffocation and the features become livid. Between the convulsions, which may follow each other rapidly, the patient is in a state of profound collapse. The principal are strychnine, prussic acid and cyanide of potassium.

In the last three groups the poison acts on the nervous system through the blood circulating in the brain.

GENERAL RULES FOR THE TREATMENT OF POISONING.

1.—When sending for a doctor, state what has occurred, whether the lips and mouth are burned, and the name of the poison if known.

2.—If breathing is failing or cannot be discerned, at once apply artificial respiration.

3.—(a) **If the lips and mouth are burned DO NOT GIVE AN EMETIC,** but an

ANTIDOTE which will neutralise the poison :—

(i) If an Acid is known to be the poison, at once give one of the following Alkalies :— Lime-water in large quantities, **or a** tablespoonful of whitening, chalk or magnesia in a tumblerful ($\frac{1}{2}$-pint) **of** water, repeated frequently.

(ii) If an Alkali is known to be the poison, at once give one of the following Acids :— Vinegar or lemon-juice or lime-juice, each diluted with an equal quantity of water, by the tumblerful.

(iii) If these antidotes are not readily available, or if it is not known whether the corrosive poison is an Acid or an Alkali, give copious draughts of cold water, or of milk. *olive oil*

(b) **Except when the lips and mouth are burned, promptly GIVE AN EMETIC**—that is, make the patient vomit and so try to get rid of the poison, by giving either :—

(i) *Mustard powder*—a tablespoonful in **a** tumblerful ($\frac{1}{2}$-pint) of lukewarm **water, or**

(ii) *Salt*—two tablespoonfuls in a tumblerful ($\frac{1}{2}$-pint) of lukewarm water.

(iii) Dirty dish water

Repeat the emetic every five minutes until vomiting occurs. If an emetic is not immediately available, induce vomiting by putting two fingers to the back of the throat.

4.—(a) In cases of corrosive poisons, after the antidote has been given, apply a hot compress to the front of the neck, and give butter, olive or salad oil or medicinal paraffin, or demulcent drinks, such as barley water or gruel; all of these tend to relieve the pain.

(b) **In cases of irritant poisons, after the emetic has acted give castor oil, two** tablespoonfuls to an adult, and two teaspoonfuls to a child. To relieve the pain give olive or salad oil or medicinal paraffin, or demulcent drinks such as barley water or gruel.

(c) **In cases of hypnotic poisons, after the emetic has been given,** if the patient threatens to go to sleep, keep him awake by walking him about and slapping his face, neck and chest with a wet towel. Give strong black coffee freely.

(d) **In cases of convulsant poisons,** the emetic can only be given and artificial respiration must only be attempted between the convulsions.

5.—In all cases give milk, raw eggs beaten up with milk or water, cream and flour beaten up together, or strong tea.

6.—Preserve any vomited matter, food or other substance suspected of being the poison. Do not wash vessels which may have contained the poison, but carefully guard them.

POISONS WHICH REQUIRE SPECIAL TREATMENT.

(a).—**Carbolic Acid (Phenol) and Lysol.** The signs and symptoms are those of corrosive acid poisoning ; the characteristic odour of the breath will aid in the detection of this poison.

TREATMENT.

1. If readily available, give half a pint of medicinal paraffin, or, if not available, Epsom or Glauber Salts, one tablespoonful in a tumblerful of milk or water.

2. Adopt the general rules which apply.

(b).—**Corrosive Sublimate (Perchloride of Mercury).** The signs and symptoms are those of an irritant poison.

TREATMENT.

1. Before the emetic give white of eggs mixed with milk or water, in unlimited quantities.

2. Adopt the general rules which apply.

(c).—**Iodine.** The signs and symptoms are those of an irritant poison, together with intense thirst ; the vomited matter may be yellow or blue.

TREATMENT.

1. Before the emetic give starch and water freely or, failing this, thin cornflour or arrowroot.

2. Adopt the general rules which apply.

(*d*).—**Phosphorus.** The signs and symptoms are those of an irritant poison.

TREATMENT.

1. Adopt the general rules which apply.

2. Give Epsom or Glauber Salts, one table-spoonful in a tumblerful of water.

Oil or fat in any form must **not** be given.

(*e*).—**Opium** and its preparations.

TREATMENT.

1. Adopt the general rules which apply.

2. After the emetic has acted give ten grains (as much as will lie on a sixpenny piece) of per-manganate of potassium; or two tablespoonfuls of Condy's fluid in a pint of water, preferably warm; repeat the dose in half an hour.

(*f*).—**Alcohol.** In the early stages the face is flushed, the eyes bloodshot and the pupils equally dilated. When the face becomes pale, the pupils dilated and fixed and the temperature of the body lowered, the patient has passed into a state of collapse and coma.

Treatment.

   1. Promote warmth of the body.
   2. Ensure rest and shelter.
   3. Adopt the general rules which apply.
   4. Give hot strong coffee.

   (g).—**Strychnine** (contained in many Vermin Killers). The signs and symptoms are a feeling of suffocation, livid features and convulsions during which the patient rests on his head and feet, and the body is arched. Between convulsions, which may follow each other rapidly, the patient is usually in a state of profound collapse.

Treatment.

   1. Between the convulsions give an emetic and perform artificial respiration.
   2. Adopt the general rules which apply.

   (h).—**Prussic Acid and Cyanide of Potassium.** The signs and symptoms are giddiness, staggering, insensibility accompanied by panting respiration, profound collapse and convulsions; in addition a smell of bitter almonds is often present. As the action of these poisons is extremely rapid, not a moment should be lost in carrying out the treatment.

TREATMENT.

1. Apply artificial respiration, even if breathing has not ceased.

2. If the patient can swallow, give freely brandy, whisky or sal volatile diluted with an equal quantity of water.

3. Dash cold water on the head and spine continuously.

4. Adopt the general rules which apply.

Salts of Lemon
_____

anhidote chalk or lime water

Chapter XV.

MISCELLANEOUS INJURIES.

SCALDS AND BURNS.

A scald is caused by moist heat, such as boiling water, steam, hot oil or tar.

A burn is caused—

(*a*) By dry heat, such as fire or a piece of hot iron.

(*b*) By a rail, wire or dynamo charged with a high tension electric current, or by lightning.

(*c*) By friction, caused, for example, by contact with a revolving wheel. (Brush-burn.)

(*d*) By a corrosive acid, such as oil of vitriol.

(*e*) By a corrosive alkali, such as caustic soda, strong ammonia, or quicklime.

The effects of a scald or burn may be a mere reddening of the skin ; blisters may be formed ; or the deeper tissues of the body may be destroyed. The clothing may adhere to the burnt skin, and its removal is impossible without further detriment to the injured part. The danger from Shock and Sepsis is very great. Every care, therefore, must be taken of the slightest burn or scald.

TREATMENT OF SCALDS, OR OF BURNS CAUSED BY DRY HEAT, ELECTRICITY OR FRICTION.

A. When medical aid or hospital is readily available.

Cover the injured part with cotton wool and bandage lightly.

B. When medical aid or hospital is not readily available.

1.—Carefully remove the clothing from the injured parts unless it sticks to the skin, when the adhering portion must be cut around carefully with clean scissors, and left in position.

2.—Do not break blisters.

3.—Immediately exclude air :—

(*a*) Place the injured part in water at the temperature of the body (98.4 degrees) until suitable dressings can be procured. A dessertspoonful of baking soda (bicarbonate of soda) to a pint of warm water will make a soothing lotion, and should be used if available. It will also serve to soak off any clothing adhering to the burn.

    (*b*) Dress the injured parts by applying strips
        of lint, linen or gauze soaked in
           (i) a fresh solution of baking soda of
               similar strength and warmth, keeping
               them moist until medical aid is
               obtained; or in
          (ii) warm strong tea, allowing them to
               dry.
    (*c*) If these are not readily available proceed
        as in 4.

4.—Cover with cotton wool or similar soft
material and bandage lightly.

5.—Give fluids freely.

**A young child, when severely scalded or
burnt,** may be placed in a warm bath of the
soothing lotion, without removing the clothes,
and kept there until medical aid is obtained,
care being taken to maintain the temperature of
the water at 98.4 degrees. This will lessen shock
and pain.

When the face is burnt, cover it with cotton
wool, lint or linen, soaked in the soothing lotion,
and keep it moist. Leave a hole for the nose and
mouth.

When a person's clothing catches fire,
approach him holding a rug, blanket, coat or
table-cover in front of yourself for protection.

Wrap it round the patient, lay him flat and so smother the flames.

If a person's clothing catches fire when alone, he should roll on the floor, smothering the flames with the nearest available wrap and call for assistance; on no account should he rush into the open air.

The use of fire-guards would prevent many calamities.

TREATMENT OF BURNS CAUSED BY A CORROSIVE ACID.

1.—If it can be obtained quickly, **bathe the part freely with an alkaline lotion,** such as a dessert-spoonful of baking soda (bi-carbonate of soda) or washing soda (carbonate of soda) in one pint of warm water. Otherwise thoroughly flood the burnt part with water, warm if immediately available.

2.—Treat as a burn.

TREATMENT OF BURNS CAUSED BY A CORROSIVE ALKALI.

1.—If the burn is caused by quicklime, brush off any that remains on the part.

2.—If it can be obtained quickly, **bathe the part freely with an acid lotion,** such as vinegar, lemon-juice or lime-juice diluted with an equal quantity of warm water. Otherwise thoroughly flood the burnt part with water, warm if immediately available.

3.—Treat as a burn.

STINGS OF PLANTS AND INSECTS.

These give rise to serious inconvenience, and in some cases grave symptoms develop.

TREATMENT.

1.—Extract the sting if present, preferably with the point of a sterilized needle.

2.—Apply freely spirit, sal volatile, a solution of baking soda (bi-carbonate of soda), washing soda (carbonate of soda) or the wet blue bag to relieve pain.

3.—Apply a dry dressing.

FROST BITE

During exposure to severe cold, parts of the body, usually the feet, fingers, nose, or ears, lose sensation and become first waxy white and afterwards congested and of a purple appearance. As sensation is lost in the part, it is often only by the remarks of bystanders that the frost-bitten person is made aware of his condition.

TREATMENT.

1.—Do not bring the patient into a warm room until, by **mild friction and the application of dry, gentle warmth,** sensation and circulation in the affected parts are restored. Neglect of this precaution may lead to death of the tissues of the frost-bitten part. Avoid the application of moisture in any form.

2.—**As soon as circulation is restored** bring the patient into a warm room.

NEEDLE EMBEDDED UNDER THE SKIN.

When a needle breaks off after penetrating the skin and disappears, take the patient and the broken piece of needle to a doctor at once. If the wound is near a joint, keep the limb at rest on a splint.

FISH-HOOK EMBEDDED IN THE SKIN.

If the hook is a large one or deeply embedded, take the patient to a doctor at once. If the hook is a small one, do not attempt to withdraw it by the way it went in, but cut off the dressing of the hook, so that only the metal is left; paint the hook and surrounding skin with an antiseptic, and then force the point onwards through the skin until the hook can be pulled out, thus making a second opening in the skin. Dress the wounds.

RUPTURE.

(Strangulated hernia)

Rupture (hernia) consists of a protrusion of the bowel through the muscular wall of the abdomen under the skin. It occurs most frequently at the groin. The signs and symptoms are a sudden swelling and pain, sometimes followed by vomiting.

TREATMENT.

1.—Lay the patient down, raise and support the head and shoulders; bend the knees and place a pillow under them.

2.—Apply ice or a cold compress to the affected part.

3.—Make no attempt to reduce the swelling.

FOREIGN BODY IN THE EYE.

1.—**Prevent the patient rubbing the eye,** tying down a child's hands if necessary.

2.—**Pull down the lower eyelid,** when, if the foreign body is seen, it can readily be removed with a camel-hair brush, or with the corner of a handkerchief twirled up and wetted with clean water.

3.—**When the foreign body is beneath the**

upper eyelid lift the lid forward, push up the lower lid beneath it and let go. The lashes of the lower lid brush the inner surface of the upper one, and may dislodge the body. Should the first attempt be unsuccessful, repeat it several times if necessary. If the foreign body is not dislodged, take the patient to a doctor as soon as possible. **When, however, medical aid cannot be had,** proceed as follows :—

    (a) Seat the patient so as to face the light, and stand behind him, steadying his head against your chest.

    (b) Place a match on the upper eyelid, half-an-inch above the edge, pressing it backwards as far as possible. Pull the upper eyelashes upwards over it, and thereby evert the eyelid.

    (c) Remove the foreign body, as in 2 above.

When a foreign body is embedded in the eyeball do not attempt to remove it, but drop medicinal paraffin or castor oil on the eyeball after pulling down the lower eyelid, close the lids, apply a soft pad of cotton wool, and secure it by a bandage tied sufficiently firmly to keep the eyeball steady.

When quicklime or other corrosive alkali is in the eye, bathe the eye with vinegar and cold water (one part in four), and treat as for a foreign body embedded in the eyeball. If vinegar is not readily obtainable, wash freely with cold water.

When oil of vitriol or other corrosive acid is in the eye bathe the eye with a solution of baking soda (a dessertspoonful in a pint of cold water) and treat as for a foreign body embedded in the eyeball.

FOREIGN BODY IN THE EAR CHANNEL.

If an insect is in the ear channel, fill the ear with olive oil, when the insect will float and may be removed. Otherwise make no attempt to treat a patient with a foreign body in the ear, but take him to a doctor as soon as possible ; attempts to remove the foreign body may lead to fatal consequences. If a child cannot be induced to keep the fingers from the ear, tie his hands down to prevent him pushing the foreign body further. Never syringe or probe the ear.

FOREIGN BODY IN THE NOSE.

Instruct the patient to breathe through the mouth. Do not interfere with the foreign body but take him to a doctor at once.

FOREIGN BODY IN THE STOMACH.

Pins, and other small sharp objects, may be accidentally swallowed. Give nothing by the mouth but take the patient to a doctor at once. Smooth objects such as coins or buttons need not cause alarm.

———————————

Chapter XVI.

ROUTINE EXAMINATION OF A PATIENT.

The First-Aider should acquire a regular and orderly method of approach to, and examination of, a patient so as to be able quickly to diagnose and efficiently to treat the condition.

Method of approach :—

1.—Approach the patient quickly and note the surroundings for any possible sources of danger or clues to diagnosis.

2.—Take first aid material with you if readily available.

3.—Detain anyone who may either afford information or be of assistance.

4.—Speak encouragingly to the patient as you approach ; warn him to lie still ; state that you are a First-Aider.

5.—Control a crowd if present, and allow the patient plenty of fresh air.

6.—Enquire the history of the accident, the exact position of any pain, and any other symptoms.

Method of Examination :—

(a) If the patient is unconscious or if the information given by him is confused and therefore unreliable, depend entirely on your own powers of observation :—

1.—Note if severe hæmorrhage is present.

2.—Note if breathing is present.

3.—If breathing is present, note whether it is slow or quick, deep or shallow, or stertorous (loud snoring and puffing of the cheeks during expiration). Note the odour of the breath. Do not assume that a person is insensible as the result of drink merely because the breath or mouth smells of alcohol. Frequently when people are feeling ill they take or are given alcoholic stimulants, after which they may become insensible, not from the drink, but from the cause that induced them to take it, for example, faintness or severe pain. Even if alcohol is the actual cause of insensibility, it must be borne in mind that the patient is therefore in a very dangerous state and must be treated accordingly.

4.—Feel the pulse by placing the first three fingers on the radial artery at the front of the patient's wrist, and pressing it lightly; the finger-tips must be half an inch away from the outer edge of the wrist on the thumb side. The pulse may be slow or quick, feeble or strong or absent altogether. If it cannot be felt, place the hand over the heart to ascertain if it beats.

5.—Note the colour of the face.

6.—Examine the head for injury; the ears, eyes and nose for hæmorrhage; and the mouth for blood, froth, burns by corrosives, and for foreign bodies.

7.—Raise the eyelids and examine the state of the pupils. In several conditions the pupils are altered; they may be both widely dilated or both minutely contracted, or, on the other hand, they may be unequal (one large and the other small). The pupils are said to be fixed when in either a bright or a shaded light no alteration takes place in their size.

8.—Examine the body and limbs for signs of fractures, dislocations, wounds; and compare the two sides of the body as to limpness.

9.—Note the condition of the skin, whether it be dry or moist, hot or cold.

(b) If, however, the patient is conscious and able to give reliable information, a detailed examination as above may be curtailed :—

1.—Examine first the position at which pain is felt, especially for dampness indicating hæmorrhage, or deformity indicating fractures or dislocations.

2.—Examine quickly for other possible injuries.

While examining the patient uncover him as little as possible since exposure increases shock.

Chapter XVII.

PREPARATION FOR RECEPTION OF ACCIDENTS.

1.—Select room.—Choose one which is easy of access, on the ground floor if possible. It should be large and airy and preferably with a fireplace which will ensure efficient ventilation. In private houses the choice is necessarily limited, but one with a cheerful sunny aspect is desirable. The patient's own room is the best if it fulfils these requirements.

2.—Clear passage and staircase of furniture and mats so far as possible.

3.—Prepare the bedroom.—Light the bedroom fire and remove all unnecessary furniture. Place the bed so that both sides are easy of access.

4.—Prepare the bed.—A single bedstead with a firm mattress (not a feather bed) should be used. If the patient has sustained a fracture of the pelvis or lower limb place transverse boards under the mattress, and have ready a bed-cradle.

Remove the upper bedclothes, place a mackintosh

or waterproof in the bed, and a draw-sheet on that portion of the bed on which the injured part will lie. Over this place a temporary blanket or sheet, aprons, brown paper or even newspapers, to keep the bed clean until the soiled clothing is removed and the patient has been attended to by the doctor.

Place hot bottles or hot bricks covered with flannel in the bed.

5.—Guard against collapse.—Have ready hot blankets, tea, coffee and other stimulants.

6.—Have ready for the doctor a small, easily moved table, basins large and small, plenty of hot and cold sterilised water, soap, nail brush, towels, cotton wool, pins, scissors, a pail to receive the dirty things, and any dressings and antiseptics available.

7.—Clean clothing for the patient should be airing by the fire, and extra bedclothes and pillows in case they should be needed.

Chapter XVIII.

TRANSPORT OF INJURED PERSONS.

(See Syllabus, page 4, Sixth Lecture.)

An injured person may be removed to shelter by the following methods :—

1. Support by a single helper.
2. Hand seats.
3. Stretcher.
4. Wheeled transport.

The method or methods adopted will depend upon the following factors :—

(*a*) The nature of the injury.
(*b*) The severity of the injury.
(*c*) The number of helpers available.
(*d*) The distance to shelter.
(*e*) The nature of the route to be traversed.

After the appropriate First Aid treatment has been given the following principles of transport must be kept in mind :—

A. The position assumed by the patient or in which he has been placed must not be disturbed unnecessarily.

G

B. Throughout the transport a careful watch must be kept on—

i. The general condition of the patient.

ii. Any dressings, tourniquets, etc., that may have been applied.

C. The transport must be safe, steady and speedy.

METHODS OF CARRYING.

If only one bearer is available—

" CRADLE."

Lift the patient by passing one of your arms beneath his two knees, and the other round his back. The arms must be passed well under before commencing to lift. This method is suitable only in the case of children or light patients.

" HUMAN CRUTCH."

Standing at his injured side, assist the patient by putting your arm round his waist, grasping the clothing at his hip and placing his arm round your neck, holding his hand with your free hand (Fig. 79).

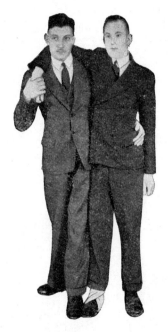

FIG. 79.—" HUMAN CRUTCH."

"PICK-A-BACK."

If the patient is conscious and able to hold on, he may be carried in the ordinary "pick-a-back" fashion.

If two or more bearers are available—

Hand Seats.

THE FOUR-HANDED SEAT.

This seat is used when the patient can assist the bearers by using one or both arms.

1.—Two bearers face each other behind the patient and grasp their left wrists with their right

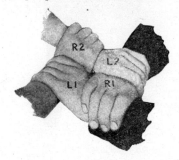

FIG. 80.—GRIP FOR FOUR-HANDED SEAT.

hands and each other's right wrists with their left hands (Fig. 80), and stoop down.

2.—The patient is instructed to place one arm round the neck of each bearer so that he may raise himself to sit on their hands and steady himself during transport.

3.—The bearers rise together and step off, the bearer on the right-hand side of the patient with the right foot, and the left-hand bearer with the left foot.

THE THREE-HANDED SEAT.

This seat is used for carrying a patient and supporting either of his lower limbs, when he is able to use one or both arms.

1.—Two bearers face each other behind the patient. For supporting the left limb the bearer on the patient's right grasps the lower end of his own left forearm with his right hand, and the lower end of the other bearer's right forearm with his left hand. The bearer on the left grasps the lower end of the first bearer's right forearm with his right hand (Fig. 81). This leaves his left hand free to support the patient's left leg. For the patient's right lower limb follow the same directions, substituting " right " for " left " and " left " for " right."—In other words, if the left leg is injured the bearer on the sound side grasps the lower end of his left forearm; if the right leg is injured, he grasps the lower end of his right forearm. The bearers stoop down.

2.—The patient is instructed to place one arm

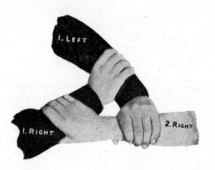

Fig. 81.—Grip for Three-Handed Seat.

round the neck of each bearer so that he may raise himself to sit on their hands and steady himself during transport.

3.—The bearers rise together and step off, the right-hand bearer with the right foot, and the left-hand bearer with the left foot.

THE TWO-HANDED SEAT.

This seat is mostly used to carry a patient who is unable to assist the bearers by using his arms.

1 —Two bearers face each other and stoop—(not

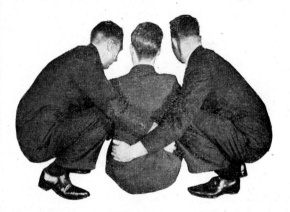

FIG. 82.
TWO-HANDED SEAT.

kneel)—one on each side of the patient. Each bearer passes his forearm nearest to the patient's head under his back just below the shoulders, and, if possible, takes hold of his clothing. They slightly raise the patient's back, and then pass their other forearms under the middle of his thighs (Fig. 82), and clasp their hands, the bearer on the left of the patient with his palm upwards and holding a folded handkerchief to prevent hurting by the finger nails; the bearer on the right of the patient with his palm downwards, as shown in Fig. 83 ("Hook-grip").

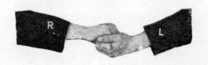

FIG. 83.—METHOD OF FORMING "HOOK-GRIP." (FRONT VIEW.)

2.—The bearers rise together and step off, the right-hand bearer with the right foot, and the left-hand bearer with the left foot (Fig. 84).

In all cases of carrying by Hand Seats the bearers walk with the cross-over step and not by side paces.

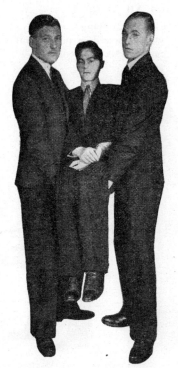

FIG. 84 —CARRYING BY TWO-HANDED SEAT.

The Fore and Aft Method.

This method of carrying (see Fig. 85) should on y be used when space does not permit of a hand seat. The bearers walk in step.

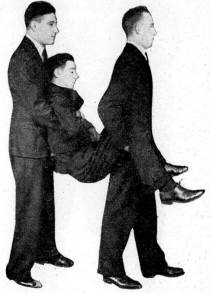

FIG. 85—FORE AND AFT METHOD.

Stretchers.

THE "FURLEY" STRETCHERS.

The "Furley" Stretchers are of two patterns, viz., "Ordinary," and "Telescopic-handled." In general principle they are alike, the component parts being designated the poles, handles, jointed traverses, runners, bed, pillow sack and slings.

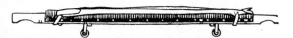

FIG. 86.—ORDINARY STRETCHER—CLOSED.

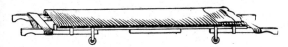

FIG. 87.—TELESCOPIC-HANDLED STRETCHER—OPEN.

The Ordinary Stretcher (Fig. 86) is 7 feet 9 inches in length, and 1 foot 10 inches wide. The bed is 6 feet in length, and the handles $10\frac{1}{2}$ inches. The height is about 6 inches. The weight is 21 to 22 lbs.

At the head of the stretcher is a canvas overlay (the pillow sack), which can be filled with straw, hay, clothing, etc., to form a pillow. The pillow sack opens at the head, and its contents can therefore be adjusted without undue disturbance of the patient. The traverses are provided with joints for opening or closing the stretcher. The Telescopic-handled pattern (Fig. 87) is similar, but the handles can be slid underneath the poles, thus reducing the length to 6 feet. This arrangement is of great value when working in confined spaces, or when a patient has to be taken up or down a narrow staircase with sharp turns. The St. John carrying sheet is also useful in similar circumstances.

When closed, the poles of the stretcher lie close together, the traverse bars being bent inwards, the canvas bed neatly folded on the top of the poles and held in position by the slings which are laid along the canvas and secured by a strap which is placed transversely at the end of each sling and passed through the large loop of the other, and round the poles and bed.

STRETCHER EXERCISES.

Based mainly on the Royal Army Medical Corps Training Manual, 1935 :—

EXERCISE No. I.

FOR FOUR BEARERS.

1.—The Instructor selects the bearers and numbers them—1, 2, 3, 4 at his discretion. Should one man be taller and stronger than the others, he should be No. 4, as he will have to bear the heavier part of the burden. All orders will be given by No. 1.

2.—" **Stand to Stretcher.** "—No. 2 places himself on the left of the stretcher, with his toes in line with the front end of the poles; No. 4 behind No. 2, with his heels in line with the rear end of the poles; No. 1 places himself on the right of the stretcher in line with No. 2, and No. 3 behind No. 1 in line with No. 4 (Fig. 88). (These are their "permanent" positions.)

3.—" **Lift Stretcher.** "—Nos. 2 and 4 stoop, grasp both handles of the poles firmly with the right hand, rise together, holding the stretcher at full extent of the arm, runners to the right.

4.—" Collect Wounded."—The squad will double by the shortest route to the patient, the leading bearers halting three paces from the head of and in line with the patient.

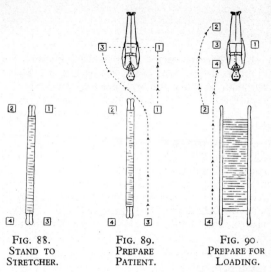

FIG. 88.
STAND TO
STRETCHER.

FIG. 89.
PREPARE
PATIENT.

FIG. 90.
PREPARE FOR
LOADING.

5.—" Lower Stretcher—Prepare Stretcher." —No. 1 proceeds to the right and No. 3 to the left of the patient, halting at his hips, and prepare him for removal (Fig. 89) ; Nos. 2 and 4 turn to the right, kneel on the left knee, unbuckle the transverse straps and place the slings on the ground beside them, separate the poles and straighten the traverses ; then each takes up a sling, doubles it on itself, slips the loop thus formed on the near handle, and places the free ends over the opposite handle, buckle uppermost. They then rise, test stretcher, arrange blankets as in Figs. 91 and 92, and proceed to the patient, taking up their positions, No. 2 opposite his knees and No. 4 opposite his shoulders as in Fig. 90, unless otherwise directed by No. 1.*

6.—" Load Stretcher."—The bearers, turning inwards together and kneeling on the left knee, will, with the exception of No. 4, pass their hands beneath the patient. (When lifting the patient from his right side, the bearers will kneel on the right knee). No. 2 supports the legs, Nos. 1 and 3 (joining hands by the " Hook-Grip ") the

---

*NOTE.—The position of the stretcher and of the bearers will be modified at the discretion of No. 1, who will be governed by the nature of the patient's injury or the surroundings.

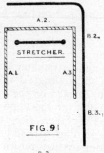

FIG. 91

There are two blankets "A" and "B," the three equal parts of each being marked A.1, A.2, A.3, and B.1, B.2, B.3. *Blanket A* is folded with its middle third A.2 over the stretcher, and one third hanging down on each side A.1 and A.3; *Blanket B* has two thirds, B.2 and B.3, hanging down on the same side.

There are now two thicknesses of blanket on the stretcher.

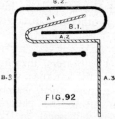

FIG. 92

A.1 is folded over B.1; A.3 remains hanging; B.2 is folded over A.1—B.3 comes right over and hangs down on the opposite side, with its centre fold B.2 over A.1.

There are now four thicknesses of blanket on the stretcher.

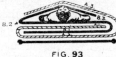

FIG. 93

" BLANKETING " A
STRETCHER.

The patient will be laid on the four thicknesses of blanket, and two thicknesses A.3 and B.3 will be folded over him.

thighs and hips, No. 4 the upper part of the trunk, passing his left hand across the patient's chest and grasping his right shoulder, and his right

No. 4.   No. 1. No. 3.   No. 2.

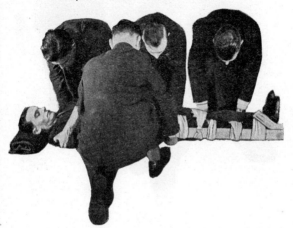

FIG. 94.
READY TO LIFT PATIENT.

arm beneath the left shoulder supporting the head (Fig. 94). In lifting the patient off the ground, special care must be taken of the injured part, No. 1 giving the necessary instructions.

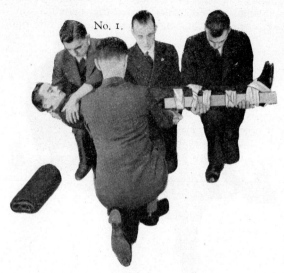

No. 4.   No. 3.   No. 2.

No. 1.

FIG. 95.
LIFTING PATIENT.

7.—" Lift."—The patient will be carefully lifted
on to the knees of Nos. 2, 3 and 4 (Fig.95). No. 1
will then disengage, rise, turn to his left, double to the
stretcher, take hold of it, left hand across, resting

the near pole on his left hip, return to the patient and place the stretcher directly beneath him (Fig. 96); then stand up and return to his former position, kneel on his left knee, join hands with No. 3, and assist in lowering the patient.

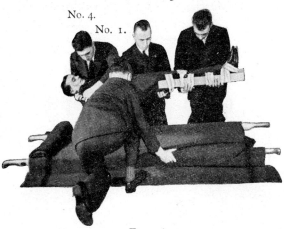

FIG. 96.
PLACING STRETCHER.

8.—"Lower."—The patient is lowered slowly and gently on to the centre of the stretcher, special

care being taken of the injured part (Fig. 97). The
bearers then disengage, cover the patient with the
two folds of blanket (A3 and B3, Fig. 93), rise,
turn to the foot end of the stretcher, and resume
their permanent positions (unless otherwise directed
by No. 1), thus :—Nos. 1 and 2 step forward and
No. 4 steps back ; No. 3 takes a side-pace to the

No. 1.   No. 3.

No. 4.   No. 2.

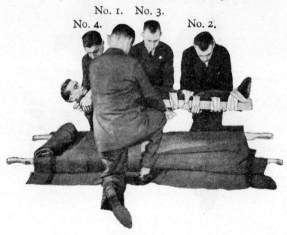

FIG. 97.
LOWERING PATIENT.

left, turns about and proceeds round the head end of the stretcher to his place on the right of the stretcher.

9.—" Lift Stretcher."—Nos. 2 and 4 stoop, grasp the doubled sling midway between the poles with the right hand and sweep it off the handles, rise, holding it at full length of the arm, buckle to the front. They then take a side-pace between the handles and place the sling over the shoulders, dividing it equally, buckle to the right. The sling should lie well below the collar of the coat behind, and in the hollow of the shoulders in front. They stoop, slip the loops over the handles, commencing with the left, and grasp both handles firmly. No. 1 will then ensure that they rise slowly together lifting the stretcher, No. 4 conforming closely to the movements of No. 2.

10.—" Adjust Slings."—Nos. 1 and 3 will turn to the left and adjust the slings of Nos. 2 and 4, and resume their permanent positions. No. 3 will collect any property belonging to the patient and, if practicable, place it on the stretcher.

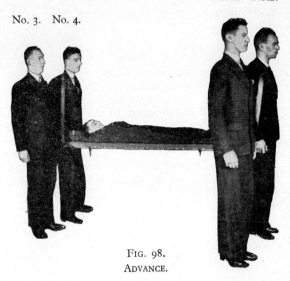

No. 1. No. 2.

No. 3. No. 4.

FIG. 98.
ADVANCE.

11.—"**Advance.**"—The bearers move off together, with a step of 20 inches, No. 4 stepping off with his right foot, the remainder of the bearers with the left foot, Nos. 2 and 4 bearers keeping their knees bent and raising their feet as little as possible.

12.—" Halt."—The bearers halt.

13.—" Lower Stretcher."—Nos. 2 and 4 slowly stoop and place the stretcher gently on the ground (No. 4 conforming to the movements of No. 2), slip the loops from the handles and stand up. They remove the slings from the shoulders, hold them as described in Order 9, take a side-pace to the left, and stand to stretcher. They then place the slings on the handles (as in Order 5) and rise together.

14.—" Unload Stretcher."—The bearers will place themselves as described for loading in Order 6.

" LIFT "—The patient, in the blankets, is lifted as described for loading.

No. 1 grasps the stretcher as described for loading, and, lifting it clear of the patient, carries it forward three paces clear of the patient's feet. He then rejoins the bearers, kneels on his left knee, joins hands with No. 3, and assists in lowering the patient to the ground. The bearers rise and resume their " permanent" positions.

15.—" Close Stretcher."—Nos. 2 and 4 turn to the right, kneel on the left knee, remove the slings and place them on the ground beside them, push in the traverses, raise the canvas, and approximate the poles, they then rise, lifting the stretcher, and face one another; place the handles of the poles between their thighs, runners to the right and fold the canvas to the right, lightly on the poles. Each takes up a sling and passes the buckle end to the other, and, holding the buckle end in the left hand, threads the transverse strap through the loop of the other sling, and buckles it tightly close to the traverse bars, keeping the sling on top. Then grasping both handles in the right hand, back of hand to the (original) right, they turn to the (original) right in a slightly stooping position, rise and turn to the left together. Nos. 1 and 3 take a side-pace to the left.

CHANGING NUMBERS.

"**Change Numbers.**"—Nos. 1 and 2 will exchange places by marching round the foot end

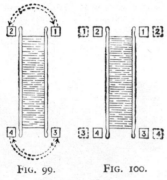

FIG. 99.   FIG. 100.

CHANGING NUMBERS.

of the stretcher and will turn about. Nos. 3 and 4 will turn about and exchange places by marching round the head end of the stretcher (Fig. 99). Each man halts in the position of the bearer whose place he has taken. The new No. 1 will take command.

NOTE.—The figures in dotted squares (**Fig. 100**) show the new positions of the old numbers.

EXERCISE No. II.

For Three Bearers.

In the event of there being only three bearers available, the stretcher will be placed at the patient's head, in the same line as his body. The bearers will then lift the patient. No. 1 kneels on the left knee on the injured side opposite the patient's

No. 3. No. 2. No. 1.

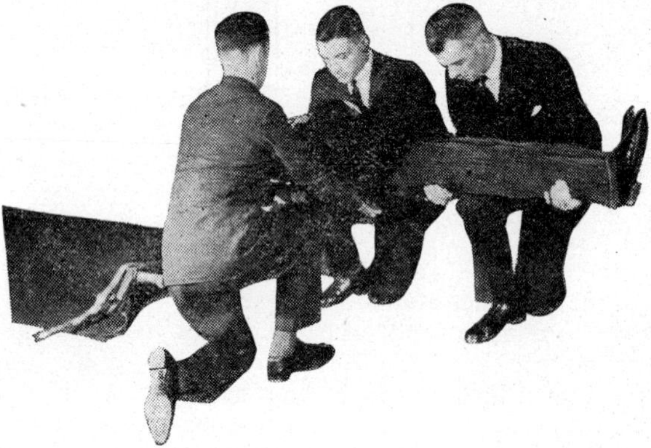

Fig. 101.
Ready to Lift Patient.

knees and passes his hands under the patient's legs;
Nos. 2 and 3 kneel on their left knees on opposite
sides of the patient, facing each other, and, passing
their hands under his shoulders and hips, lock their

No. 3.   No. 2.   No. 1.

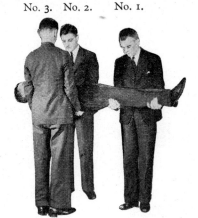

Fig. 102.

Patient Lifted.

fingers by the hook-grip. On the command
" Lift " the bearers will rise to the erect position,
and, moving by side-paces, carry him head foremost
over the foot end of the stretcher, the horizontal

position of his body being maintained throughout the movement, and lower him carefully on to the folded blankets. When unloading, the patient will be lifted and carried head foremost over the head end of the stretcher (see Figs. 101 and 102).

EXERCISE No. III.

FOR USE IN MINES AND NARROW CUTTINGS WHERE TWO MEN ONLY CAN BE ENGAGED.

Nos. 1 and 2 will carefully place the stretcher in a line with the injured man's body, the foot of the stretcher being, if possible,* close to his head.

No. 2 places his feet one on each side of the patient between his body and arms, the toe of each foot as near the armpits as possible. He then stoops down and passes his hands between the sides of the chest and the arms underneath the shoulders, and locks the fingers. No. 1 straddles across the patient's legs, placing his right foot, with the toe turned outwards, a little below the patient's knees, and with the toe of the left foot close to the heel of No. 2; he then stoops down,

---

*It is not advisable to be too particular as to the head or foot of a stretcher in a mine, as it would probably be quite impossible to reverse it.

passes the left hand under the patient's thighs and
the right hand under the patient's calves. If the
patient's arms are uninjured he may put them
round the neck of No. 2, and by this means greatly

No. 2. No. 1.

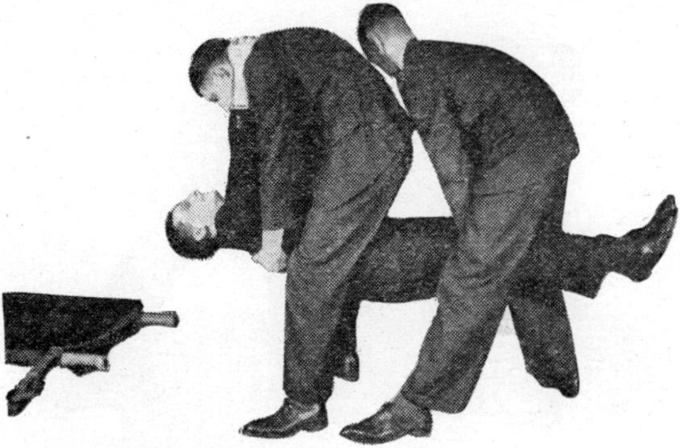

Fig. 103.
MOVING FORWARD.

assist him in lifting. If the patient is unconscious,
fold his arms across his chest.

When both are ready, No. 1 will give the order
"Lift and move forward." The patient is then
to be slowly lifted, just sufficiently to allow his

body to clear the stretcher. Both bearers will
slowly and gradually move the patient forward.
No. 2 by very short steps, No. 1 by bending his
body forward as much as he can *without moving*

No. 2.   No. 1.

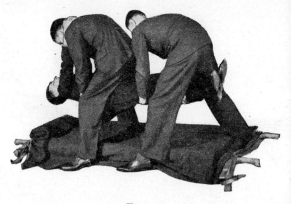

FIG. 104.
LOWERING PATIENT.

his feet (Fig. 103). No. 1 now gives the order
"**Halt,**" whereupon No. 2 remains steady, and
No. 1 advances his right foot to his left, and again
advances his left foot till the toe touches the heel of

No. 2. No. 1 then gives the order " **Advance**," when the patient will again be moved forward. These movements are to be repeated until the patient is over the stretcher, when he is to be gently lowered (Fig. 104).

IMPROVISED STRETCHERS.

Stretchers may be improvised as follows :—

1.—Turn the sleeves of two or three coats inside out; pass two strong poles through them; button the coats. The poles may be kept apart by strips of wood lashed to the poles at both ends of the bed formed by the coats.

2.—Make holes in the bottom corners of one or two sacks and pass stout poles through them, keeping the poles apart as in 1.

3.—Tie broad bandages at intervals to two poles in the manner described for raising a patient with a fracture of the spine (see pages 74 and 75).

4.—Spread out a rug, piece of sacking, tarpaulin, or a strong blanket, and roll two stout poles up in the sides. Two bearers stand on each side and grasp the middle of the covered pole with one hand, and near the end with the other. They walk sideways.

5.—A hurdle, broad piece of wood, or shutter may be used; rugs, clothing, hay, straw, etc., should be placed on it, and covered with a piece of stout cloth or sacking; the latter is useful in taking the patient off the stretcher.

Always test an improvised stretcher before use.

CARRIAGE OF STRETCHERS.

As a general rule carry the patient feet foremost.

The exceptions are :—

   (a) When going up hill with a patient whose lower limbs are not injured.

   (b) When going down hill with a patient whose lower limbs are injured.

   (c) When carrying a stretcher upstairs; an extra helper should assist at the lower end, so as to raise it and keep the stretcher nearly horizontal.

TO CROSS A DITCH.

The stretcher should be lowered with its foot one pace from the edge of the ditch. Nos. 1 and 2 bearers then descend. The stretcher is now advanced, Nos. 1 and 2 in the ditch supporting the front end while the other end rests on the edge of the ground above. Nos. 3 and 4 now descend. All the bearers now carry the stretcher to the opposite side and the foot of the stretcher is made to rest on the edge of the ground, while the head is supported by Nos. 3 and 4 in the ditch. Nos. 1 and 2 climb out. The stretcher is lifted forward on the ground above, and rests there while Nos. 3 and 4 climb up.

To Cross a Wall.

The stretcher is lowered with the foot about one pace from the wall; the bearers then stand to stretcher, Nos. 2 and 4 on the left, Nos. 1 and 3 on the right. They turn inwards, stoop down, grasp the poles with both hands; they rise slowly, lifting the stretcher, holding it level at the full extent of the arms. Then by side-paces advance to the wall, raise the stretcher and lift it on to the wall, so that the front runners are just over the wall. No. 2 then crosses the wall and takes hold of the front handles; No. 1 then crosses the wall, they grasp the poles, lift the foot of the stretcher; all the bearers then advance and lift the rear runners over the wall, resting the rear handles on the wall; No. 4 then crosses the wall and takes hold of the left pole, No. 3 then crosses the wall and takes hold of the right pole. The bearers then advance until the stretcher is clear of the wall. The stretcher is then lowered to the ground.

To Load an Ambulance.

The stretcher will be lowered with its foot or head one pace from the end of the ambulance, according to the patient's desire to travel feet or head first.

The bearers will now stand to stretcher.

"**Load.**"—The bearers turn inwards, stoop, grasp the poles of the stretcher, hands wide apart, palms uppermost; they rise slowly, lifting the stretcher, holding it level at the full extent of the arms. They then take a side-pace to the ambulance, raising the stretcher evenly to the level of the compartment to be loaded. The front bearers place the runners in the grooves and then assist the rear bearers to slide the stretcher into its place and secure it. If slings have been used, they should be kept with their stretcher.

Many ambulances are provided with upper and lower berths. In such cases the upper berths should be loaded first, beginning on the off-side.

To Unload an Ambulance.

Two bearers will take hold of the handles at the rear and gently withdraw the stretcher. As it is withdrawn, the other two will take hold of the handles at the front, and, taking the weight, lower it to the full extent of the arms; then by side-paces march clear of the ambulance, lower the stretcher to the ground, and take up their "permanent" positions.

LIFTING INTO BED.

The stretcher is lowered at the side of the bed. The bearers take positions as for unloading stretcher, Nos. 2, 3 and 4 being on the side furthest from the bed. The patient is unloaded on to the knees of Nos. 2, 3 and 4. No. 1 will disengage and remove the stretcher (this may be done by pushing it under the bed). He then joins hands with No. 3. All the bearers rise to a standing position, supporting the patient on their forearms. No. 1 disengages and goes to the patient's head, and supports it. All bearers then step forward and gently place the patient on the bed. If the bed is narrow and there is room, the stretcher may be placed on the floor with the head close to the foot of the bed. The injured person may then be lifted over the foot and placed on the bed.

———————

QUESTIONS.

The numerals indicate the pages where the answers may be found.

CHAPTER I.

FRONTISPIECE.

When describing the body how is it supposed to be placed?

If a person raises his arm above his head, which is considered to be the upper part of that limb? (Answer: The shoulder)

What is the middle line of the body?

CHAPTER II.

CHAPTER III.

CHAPTER IV. ✓

PRACTICE

CHAPTER VII.

CHAPTER VIII.

The **Student** should practise placing supposed patients in a proper position for the arrest of hæmorrhage (see pages 104, etc.), folding firm pads, **tying** hard knots in bandages to form a tourniquet (111), and the application of pressure at all the pressure points shown in the frontispiece, at various points on the forehead and scalp, and on the palm of the hand. Pressure should be digital, or by pad and bandage as directed in the text.

CHAPTER X.

CHAPTER XI.

CHAPTER XII.

CHAPTER XIII.

CHAPTER XIV.

CHAPTER XVI.

CHAPTER XVII.

CHAPTER XVIII.

INTRODUCTION TO APPENDICES.

The Textbook of the Association deals primarily with First Aid rendered by an individual at the scene of the accident with such materials as may be at hand, as distinct from "organised" First Aid as practised by First Aid units trained to work together and equipped with suitable appliances.

For the benefit of First-Aiders who have opportunities of practising together, who are equipped with suitable material and appliances and have not to rely on improvisation, some additional information is included in the Appendices which follow. They will be of special value to members of the Technical Reserves for the Medical Services of the Forces of the Crown found by the St. John Ambulance Brigade, namely, Voluntary Aid Detachments, Royal Naval Auxiliary Sick Berth Reserve and the Military Hospitals Reserve, and to those in charge of First Aid rooms.

APPENDIX I.

CARBON-DIOXIDE AND ITS USE IN ARTIFICIAL RESPIRATION.

Carbon-dioxide is recognised as a powerful stimulant to respiration and where available should be applied at the earliest possible moment to the mouth and nose, preferably through a mask. The gas is applied for three minutes and left off for three minutes until respiration begins. It may be used alone or in conjunction with oxygen, according to the apparatus available. It must be realised that the gas can be drawn into the lungs only while artificial respiration is being performed.

APPENDIX II.

TANNIC ACID TREATMENT OF BURNS AND SCALDS.

The application of a 2 per cent. tannic acid solution (3 heaped teaspoonfuls of tannic acid powder in a pint of sterile water) to burnt and scalded areas has proved a highly efficient method of treatment, the firm coagulum which results being an ideal protection.

It is used in the three following methods :—

1.—Tannic Acid Spray. A freshly made 2 per cent. tannic acid solution is sprayed on the affected area and allowed to dry, followed by successive applications until a firm coagulum is formed. Radiant heat hastens the drying.

2.—Tannic Acid Tablets. Tannic acid, gr. $17\frac{1}{2}$; perchloride of mercury, gr. $\frac{1}{2}$; boric acid, gr. 1.

The tablet is crushed to a powder between two spoons and added to 2 ounces of warm water, making a 2 per cent. solution. Gauze is soaked in the solution and applied to the burnt area in successive layers up to about six, depending on the size of the area affected.

3.—Tannic Acid Jelly. Tannic acid may be used in the form of jelly which is spread freely on gauze, applied to the injured part and kept in position by a bandage.

Care should be taken that the operator's hands are thoroughly washed and rinsed in antiseptic, that blisters are carefully removed with sterile forceps and scissors, that the dressing is in complete apposition to the affected part, and the coagulum or dressing covered by a bandage.

Appendix III.

The Thomas Splint.

This splint (which is named not after the famous hospital in London, but after the eminent surgeon, the late Mr. H. O. Thomas), may be used (a) for all fractures of the thigh-bone except where there is an extensive wound in the upper part of the thigh or buttock against which the splint would press and cause pain; (b) for any fracture about the knee-joint and bones of the leg; (c) in certain cases of extensive wounds of the fleshy part of the leg or thigh.

Outfit.

For practising the application of the splint the following outfit is desirable :—

Thomas Splint.

Stretcher suspension bar.

Reversible stirrup (Sinclair's).

Stick or 6 in. nail for Spanish windlass.

Flannelette bandage, 3 yards long by 3 inches wide.

Five flannelette bandage slings and 5 safety pins.

Five triangular bandages.

Some loose woven bandages and wool.

Two pieces of Gooch splinting about 8 inches by 6 inches.

A stretcher. (Trestles on which the stretcher may be placed are convenient when practising.)

Three blankets.

To form the slings mentioned above, five pieces of flannelette bandage, approximately 30—36 inches in length are taken and folded into two. The loop ends are pinned over the inner bar of the splint, rolled up and secured in position by short ties of loose woven bandage.

PERSONNEL.

A team for the purpose of practice usually consists of four First-Aiders, who may be numbered 1, 2, 3, and 4, and a patient; but three or even two are sufficient.

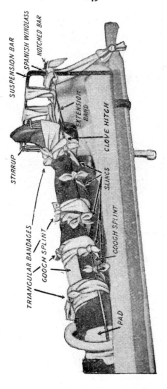

SUSPENSION BAR
SPANISH WINDLASS
NOTCHED BAR
STIRRUP
EXTENSION BAND
CLOVE HITCH
TRIANGULAR BANDAGES
GOOCH SPLINT
GOOCH SPLINT
SLINGS
GOOCH SPLINT
PAD

FIG. 105.

THE THOMAS SPLINT.

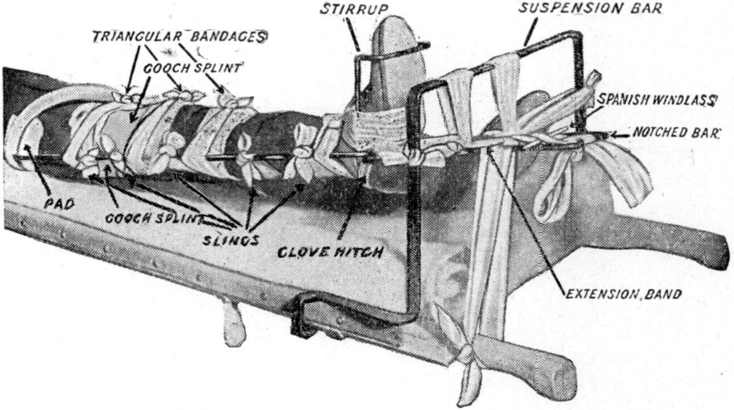

250

SUSPENSION BAR

SPANISH WINDLASS

NOTCHED BAR

EXTENSION BAND

STIRRUP

CLOVE HITCH

TRIANGULAR BANDAGES

GOOCH SPLINT

SLINGS

GOOCH SPLINT

PAD

FIG. 106.

THE THOMAS SPLINT.

Drill.

The application of the Thomas Splint can most conveniently be taught as a drill.

1. **Prepare Stretcher.**—Nos. 1 and 3 proceed to the patient and cover him with a blanket : Nos. 2 and 4 prepare the stretcher as described on pages 206 and 207 (Figs. 90–93).

2. **Hand Extension.**—No. 3 places himself at the foot of the patient facing him and opposite the injured limb. Keeping the arms straight, he grasps the heel of the boot with his right hand and the toe with his left, and, keeping the foot vertical, exerts a steady pull. No. 4 steadies and supports the injured limb above and below the seat of fracture.

3. **Apply Splint.**—No. 1 threads the ring of the splint over the boot (pointed end of ring outwards), No. 3 removing and re-applying each hand in turn to permit of this being done. While No. 4 continues to support the limb at the seat of fracture, No. 1 passes the splint up the limb until its further passage is stopped by the buttock. The notched bar must be kept horizontal.

4. **Clove Hitch.**—No. 2 takes three yards of flannel bandage and makes a clove hitch in such a way as to leave one end about six inches longer than

the other and a double loop about ten inches in diameter. This loop is applied over the boot with the ends on the outer side of the ankle : to allow of this being done No. 3, still carrying out hand extension, again removes and re-applies one hand at a time. The long end of the bandage is taken under the instep of the boot, up on the inner side of the ankle, threaded through the loop of the hitch and turned down outside the loop. These two ends of the bandage, one on either side of the ankle, are for use as extension bands when permanent extension takes the place of hand extension.

5. Fix Leg.

(a) The extension bands are tied round the notched bar as follows :—the outer extension band is passed over and under the bar, round the notch, drawn taut, and held over to the opposite side. The inner band is passed under and over the bar, then also round the notch, so that it crosses the first band and prevents it slipping. The two are tied off by a half bow. No. 3 may now release his hold.

(b) The notched bar is now placed on some object, such as an empty petrol tin turned on its side, so as to keep the limb well raised from the ground. No. 4 will continue to steady and support the limb.

(c) **The** middle sling is tied off over the outer **bar** behind the knee, No. 4 keeping the knee slightly **bent.**

(d) The slings behind the ankle and calf **are** tied off so that the leg is now supported in a shallow **trough** with the long bars of the splint level with the centre of the leg.

(e) To prevent the leg rising off the splint, **a** narrow bandage is placed across the leg just below the knee ; the ends are carried down between the leg and the splint, crossed behind, brought up outside the bars and tied off on the front of the leg.

The lower limb is thus fixed in a position of extension, and it may be moved freely without causing pain to the patient or damage to the injured part.

6. **Dress Wound.**—A wound, if present, **is** dressed in accordance with the general rules.

7. **Gooch Splinting.**—These or other well-padded cardboard splints may be applied (over **the** dressings, if any), one piece is placed behind **the** limb and secured by tying off the remaining **two** slings. The other piece is placed in front of **the** thigh, care being taken to avoid pressure on **the** knee-cap. The dressing and the splints are kept

firmly in position by two narrow bandages applied as follows :—

The centre of each bandage is placed near each end of the front piece of Gooch splinting. The ends are taken down between the limb and the side bars of the splint, crossed behind and then brought up on the outside of the bars and tied in front of the limb.

8. **Stirrup and Figure of Eight.**—The stirrup is sprung on to the splint (care being taken to keep it clear of the extension bands) and pressed upwards until the horizontal bar rests lightly against the sole of the boot, thus preventing lateral movement of the foot. A narrow bandage is applied in the following manner to form a figure of eight. The centre of the bandage is placed under the sole of the boot. The ends are brought forward, crossed, taken down behind the ankle, crossed again, brought up outside the bars and tied off in front of the limb.

9. **Spanish Windlass.**—Except in the case of a compound fracture when the bone protrudes, the extension bands are tightened and a small piece of wood or a nail may be introduced to increase the tension by twisting up as required.

10. **Pad in Ring.**—A pad of cotton wool is placed inside the ring on the outer side of the

thigh to act as a wedge and so prevent undue movement.

11. **Suspension Bar.**—This is fitted to the stretcher with the grips away from the foot end, and with its horizontal part one hand's breadth in front of the foot.

The splint is slung about one hand's breadth from the horizontal iron of the suspension bar by bandages tied to the splint bars. It is also tied to the vertical irons of the suspension bar to prevent lateral movement; to prevent vertical movement of the splint, a narrow bandage is passed round the outer side of the splint below the foot and tied off to the handle of the stretcher.

12. **Cover Patient.**—Hot water bottles are applied and the blankets adjusted as described in Fig. 93 (page 208).

The patient is now ready for removal to shelter

Appendix IV.

THE ROLLER BANDAGE AND ITS APPLICATION.

The Roller Bandage.

Roller bandages are made of woven cotton, domette, flannel, or of other suitable material. They are of various widths for different parts of

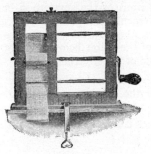

Fig. 107.—Roller Bandage Machine.

the body, and are usually 6 yards in length. They may be rolled by hand or by means of a machine (Fig. 107). When a bandage is partly unrolled the roll is called the head, and the unrolled part the free end.

Uses of the Roller Bandage.

Roller bandages are used :—

1. To retain splints or dressings in position.
2. To afford support.
3. To make pressure and so reduce or prevent swelling.
4. To drive blood from the part of the body bandaged, as in the case of extreme collapse from hæmorrhage.

General Rules for Application.

1. See that the bandage is tightly and evenly rolled before attempting to use it.
2. Apply the outer side of the free end to the part.
3. Never allow more than a few inches of the bandage to be unrolled at a time.
4. Bandage from below upwards, and from within outwards, over the front of a limb.
5. Apply each layer of the bandage so that it covers two-thirds of the preceding one.
6. Apply the bandage firmly and evenly, but not tightly enough to stop the circulation. If the edges turn up on passing the hand over them, the bandage is too loose. If, after the bandage is taken off, red lines are seen, it has not been evenly applied.
7. Fix the bandage securely when finished.

I

Methods of Application.

There are four principal methods of applying the roller bandage :—

1. **The simple spiral,** which is made by encircling the part with the bandage several times.

This should only be used when the part to be bandaged is of uniform thickness, as, for instance, the finger, or wrist and a short portion of the forearm above it.

2. **The reverse spiral,** which is made by a number of spiral turns in which the bandage is reversed downwards upon itself at each circuit of the limb.

This is used in bandaging parts of the limbs where owing to their varying thickness it is impossible to make a simple spiral lie properly (see Fig. 116).

3. **The figure of 8,** which is applied by passing the bandage obliquely round the limb, alternately upwards and downwards, the loops resembling the figure 8.

It is used for bandaging at or in the neighbourhood of a joint such as the knee or elbow. It may also be used instead of a reverse spiral for a limb.

4. **The spica,** which is a modified figure of 8 used for bandaging the shoulder, groin or thumb (see Figs. 112 and 113).

When the methods of bandaging are understood, no difficulty should arise in covering any part of the body. The points to which attention should be directed are evenness and firmness of application rather than a completed bandage corresponding exactly with the illustration. It will, in fact, be found that differently shaped limbs require slight modifications of the bandage.

No matter what is the actual position of a person, for purposes of description the body is supposed to be erect with the arms hanging by the side and the palms of the hands directed forwards.

APPLICATION TO VARIOUS PARTS.

Capeline Bandage for Head.—Take two $2\frac{1}{2}$-inch bandages and join the free ends. Standing behind the patient, who should be seated, apply the join to the middle of the forehead just above the eyebrows, heads of the bandage inwards. The bandage in the right hand is called the vertical bandage, and that in the left hand is called the horizontal bandage. Bring both rolls to the back of the head and cross them (Fig. 108). Carry the vertical bandage forwards over the head, and the horizontal bandage round the head and over the vertical bandage in front. (Fig. 109 shows the

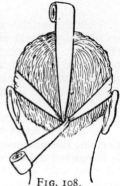

vertical bandage carried twice forwards and once backwards.) Continue to pass the vertical bandage backwards and forwards, each time a little to the left and right alternately, locking it with the horizontal bandage. Finally, pass the horizontal bandage twice round the head, and pin in front (Fig. 110).

FIG. 108.

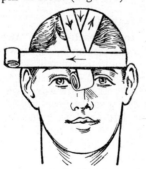

FIG. 109.

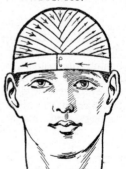

FIG. 110.

FIGS. 108-110.—CAPELINE BANDAGE FOR HEAD.

Simple Spiral for the Fingers.—*Width of bandage*, 1 inch. *Course.*—From inner to outer side of front of wrist, a sufficient length being left for tying ; across back of hand to inner side of finger to be first bandaged (taking the fingers in order from the little finger side), by one spiral to root of finger nail ; round finger by simple spirals ; thence to root of little finger and round wrist, continuing to the next finger, if necessary. When completed tie to free end left for the purpose (Fig. 111).

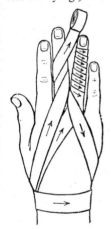

FIG. 111.
SIMPLE SPIRAL FOR
THE FINGERS.

Spica for the Thumb.—*Width of bandage*, 1 inch. *Course.*—Across front of wrist from inner to outer side ; up between thumb and finger by one spiral to root of thumb nail ; simple turn round thumb ; diagonally across back of thumb and hand to wrist ; continue by figure of 8 round thumb and wrist until the thumb is covered. Finish by a turn round wrist and secure (Figs. 112 and 113).

Bandage for the Hand.—*Width of Bandage,*
2 or 2½ inches. *Course.*—From between thumb
and finger across back of hand, front of wrist

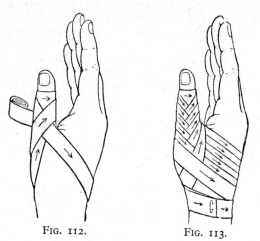

FIG. 112.   FIG. 113.

FIGS. 112, 113.—SPICA FOR THE THUMB.

and back of hand to fourth finger nail; once
round fingers (Fig. 114). Figure of 8 round hand

and wrist. Repeat figures of 8 until the hand is covered, then round wrist and secure (Fig. 115).

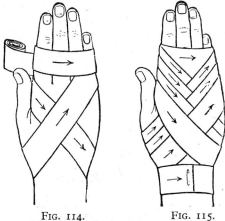

FIG. 114.   FIG. 115.
FIGS. 114, 115.—BANDAGE FOR THE HAND.

Reverse Spiral for the Forearm.—*Width of bandage,* 2 or 2½ inches. *Course.*—Across front of wrist from inner to outer side ; across back of hand to first joint of little finger ; across front of fingers ; to inner then outer side of wrist.

Repeat once. Two or three simple spirals round wrist. Reverse spirals on forearm and secure (Figs. 116 and 117).

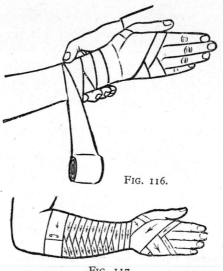

FIG. 116.

FIG. 117.

FIGS. 116, 117.—REVERSE SPIRAL FOR THE FOREARM.

The figure of 8 bandage, as for the leg (see page 269 and Fig. 130), may be applied instead of the spiral.

Figure of 8 for Elbow, Knee and Ankle.—
Width of bandage, 3 inches. *Course.*—Round
the joint and then figure of 8 alternately above
and below joint (Figs. 118 and 119). Secure.

Spica for the Shoulder (left).—*Width of
bandage,* 3 inches. *Course.*—Secure the free end
round the arm. Thence from inner side of left

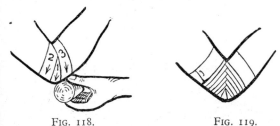

FIG. 118.   FIG. 119.

FIGS. 118, 119.—FIGURE OF 8 BANDAGE FOR ELBOW,
KNEE AND ANKLE.

arm, over the front of the arm, across the back,
under the right armpit, across the chest to the
outer side of the arm, across the back of the arm
(Fig. 120). Repeat until the part is sufficiently
covered and secure (Fig. 121).

Bandage for the Breast (right).—*Width of
bandage,* 3 inches. *Course.*—From left side of

1*

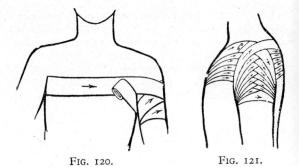

FIG. 120.   FIG. 121.

FIGS. 120, 121.—SPICA FOR THE SHOULDER.

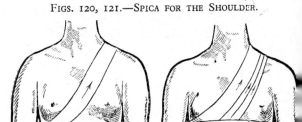

FIG. 122.   FIG. 123.

FIGS. 122, 123.—BANDAGE FOR THE BREAST.

back of waist ; round waist ; under right breast ; over left shoulder to right side of waist (Fig. 122), round waist ; repeat until the breast is sufficiently covered and supported (Fig. 123). Secure.

Bandage for Both Breasts.—*Width of bandage*, **3** inches. *Course.*—From right side of back of waist, round waist, up over front of left shoulder to right side of waist, round waist, over

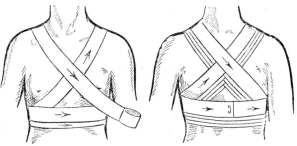

FIG. 124.   FIG. 125.

FIGS. 124, 125.—BANDAGE FOR BOTH BREASTS.

back of right shoulder to left side of waist, and round waist (Fig. 124). Repeat alternately over the left and right shoulders until both breasts are covered and supported (Fig. 125). Secure.

Spica for (right) Groin or Hip.—*Width of bandage*, **3** inches. *Course.*—Two turns round the thigh to fix the bandage. From fork to crest of right hip; across loins to left hip; thence to outer side of and behind right thigh. Repeat until the groin is sufficiently covered and secure (Figs. 126 and 127).

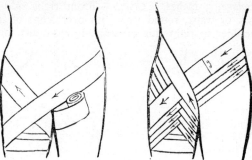

FIG. 126.   FIG. 127.
FIGS. 126, 127.—SPICA FOR GROIN OR HIP.

Bandage for the Foot.—*Width of bandage,* 2½ *inches.* *Course.*—From inner side of ankle, over foot to root of fifth toe; round foot; two or three reverse spirals round foot; figures of 8 round the ankle and foot until the part is sufficiently covered; once round ankle, and secure (Figs. 128 and 129).

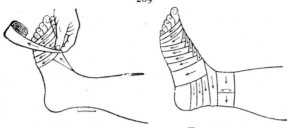

FIG. 128.   FIG. 129.
FIGS. 128, 129.—BANDAGE FOR THE FOOT.

Figure of 8 Bandage for the Leg.—*Width of bandage*, 3 inches.   *Course.*—From inner side of ankle to outer side of foot, round foot; round ankle; again round foot and ankle; and thence up the limb by ascending figure of 8, each layer covering the previous one by two-thirds (Fig. 130).   Secure.

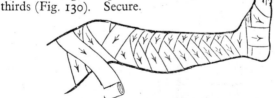

FIG. 130.—FIGURE OF 8 FOR THE LEG.

The reverse spiral, as for the forearm, may be applied instead.

Bandage for a Broken Collar-bone.

1. Place in the armpit a pad, about 2 inches thick and 4 inches across.

2. Pass the end of a 4-inch bandage round the upper part of the arm to form a loop, and secure with a safety pin.

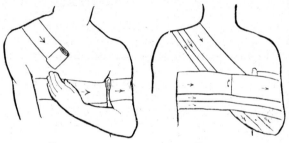

FIG. 131.   FIG. 132.
FIGS. 131, 132.—BANDAGE FOR A BROKEN COLLAR-BONE.

3. Carry the bandage across the patient's back a little below the armpits to draw the shoulder back, and continue it round the chest to the armpit on the injured side.

4. Raise the forearm well up.

5. Carry the bandage diagonally across the back and over the uninjured shoulder (Fig. 131) and

round the elbow three times to raise the shoulder and support the forearm.

6. Pass the bandage three times round the body and lower end of the arm to lever out the shoulder.

7. Secure with a safety pin (Fig. 132).

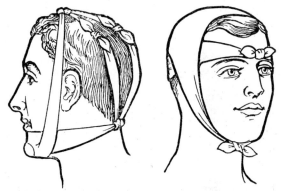

FIG. 133.—BANDAGE FOR THE JAW.

FIG. 134.—BANDAGE FOR THE HEAD.

Bandage for the Jaw.—Take one yard and a half of a 3-inch bandage. Cut a small hole in the centre, and tear the bandage from each end down the middle to within $1\frac{1}{2}$ inches of the hole, thus producing a bandage with four tails. Apply as shown in Fig. 133.

Bandage for any part of the Head.—To make the bandage, take a piece of calico about 6 inches wide and 2 feet 6 inches long. Tear the bandage down the middle from each end, leaving about 12 inches untorn. Apply as Fig. 134. This bandage, having four tails, may be applied on the same principle to the forehead or dome of the head.

MANY-TAILED BANDAGES.

These bandages may be made of domette, flannel, linen or other suitable material.

A piece of material long enough to go one and a half times round the limb, and in width sufficient to cover the dressing on the wound, may be torn from each end in parallel strips of equal width towards the centre, which remains undivided : the strips must be equal to each other in width, which will vary from 2 to 4 inches according to the part to be bandaged.

An alternative method of making the many-tailed bandage is to lay strips of suitable material parallel to each other, each overlapping one-third of the preceding one : the strips may then be

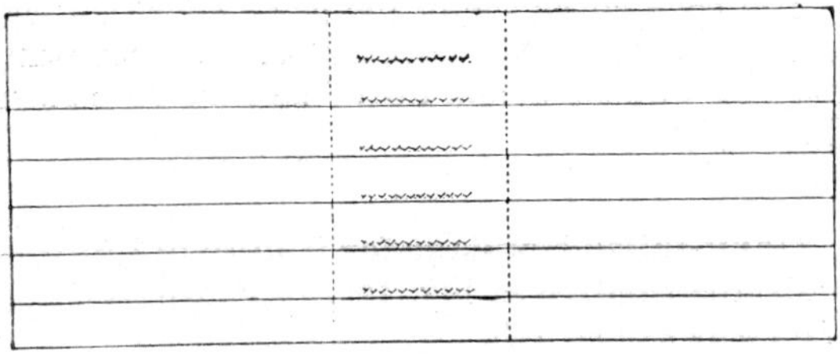

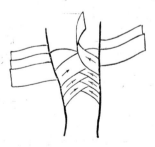

Fig. 135.—Many-tailed Bandage.

sewn together for a short distance on either side
of their centres or to a similar piece of material
laid across the centres of the strips (Fig. 135).

Fig. 136.—Many-tailed Bandage.

The chief advantage of the many-tailed bandage is that a wound can be examined or a dressing changed without undue disturbance of the patient (Fig. 136).

Many-tailed Bandage for Stump of Limb.—
Make the bandage as Fig. 137, from 3-inch calico, and apply as Fig. 138.

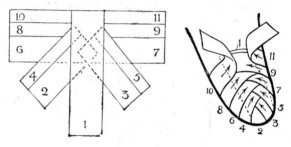

FIG. 137.   FIG. 138.

FIGS. 137, 138.—MANY-TAILED BANDAGE FOR STUMP OF LIMB.

Appendix V.

FIRST AID AND AMBULANCE AT FACTORIES AND WORKSHOPS.

At the request of the Factory Department of the Home Office, and to assist in making known the several very important First Aid Orders issued by the Home Office under the " Police, Factories, &c. (Miscellaneous Provisions) Act, 1916," the following slightly condensed extract from the official pamphlet, " First Aid and Ambulance at Factories and Workshops," is affixed to the Association's text book for the First Aid course of instruction.

Organization.

If the full benefits of First Aid and Ambulance are to be obtained, their organization must be carried out in such a manner as to ensure the co-operation of the workers. There is no side of industrial life where the interests of employers and employed are more closely identified, and where combined efforts towards improvement work more for mutual benefit.

Supervision is essential, and some person or persons must be made responsible for the smooth and satisfactory working of the organization throughout the factory, and as First Aid is so closely allied with safety, it would seem appropriate to delegate to members of any Safety Committee established at the works, the responsibility for the efficient carrying out of First Aid and Ambulance arrangements. To this Committee would fall the duties of considering suggestions regarding the adequacy of the provision made. It would also undertake arrangements for the training of persons in First Aid and the appointment of an appropriate number of them to be responsible for the First Aid Boxes.

The benefits of an effective First Aid and Ambulance service may be summarised as follows :—

Suffering is alleviated.

The workman who has met with a slight accident is enabled to return to work almost immediately in comfort and with a sense of security.

Minor accidents are prevented from developing into serious injuries as a result of septic infection or blood poisoning. Experience shows that it is not always a severe accident that in the end proves the most serious.

The loss of a limb or even of life has ensued from an apparently trivial, but neglected, injury.

The recovery of the workman and his return to work after a severe accident may be materially expedited.

The Home Office has statutory power to make Orders requiring the provision of Ambulance and First Aid arrangements at any specified works or class of works, and several Orders for different classes of work are already in force. These Orders differ somewhat according to circumstances, but are based on one general scheme comprising :—

1. **First Aid Boxes.**
   (a) For the treatment of minor injuries.
   (b) For preliminary treatment of more serious cases, e.g., hæmorrhage, fractures, unconsciousness, etc., before medical help is available.

2. **Central Ambulance Room** under the charge of a qualified nurse or other person trained in First Aid. This will be the main centre of treatment in the works, serving in particular for the preliminary treatment of the more serious cases and also for any subsequent treatment that may be required in cases dealt with at the First Aid Boxes.

First Aid Boxes.

Number and Position of First Aid Boxes. It is essential that First Aid to be successful shall be rendered immediately, and First Aid Boxes should therefore be provided in such numbers and positions as to be within easy reach of every worker. The Home Office Orders prescribe a minimum number, which is one box to every 150 persons. The best position for a First Aid Box is in the work-room itself.

Equipment of First Aid Boxes.—The equipment of the First Aid Boxes as specified in the Orders varies according to the nature of the injuries likely to occur in the particular industry or process, but, generally speaking, it consists of a supply of sterilised finger, hand and large size dressings, iodine solution, a bottle of eye drops and sterilised cotton wool, together with a copy of the First Aid leaflet issued by the Factory Department, which gives suggestions for the treatment of minor injuries. *It is best that the equipment of a First Aid Box should in most cases be limited to the articles above specified ;* cases have been brought to the notice of the Factory Department where boxes have been supplied with equipment of a quite unnecessarily elaborate character. Where, however, no ambulance room is provided, it is desirable to provide in one or more of the boxes or in a small cupboard in a central position the following additional appliances : scissors, safety pins, sal volatile and measure glass, a tourniquet, splints, slings, roller bandages, an additional supply of wool and a roll of plaster (1 inch wide), and also, in places where burns are likely to occur, a supply of sterilised burn dressings. A stretcher is also advisable.

Protection and Use of Dressings.—Dressings must be sterilised (subjected to heat to destroy any germs, and not merely impregnated with an antiseptic), but must also be kept sterile. Each dressing should therefore be in a separate packet carefully sealed, complete in itself, and so packed that it will not matter whether or not the hands of the worker who applies it are dirty. All that is necessary is to avoid touching that part of the dressing which is to be placed upon the wound.

Waterproof Plaster.—Waterproof plaster to cover dressings is required in Dyeing and Tanning Works where solutions of bichromate of potassium are used, in order to prevent the solution in which the worker's hands are immersed from saturating the dressings and attacking the wound. To be successful the plaster must be applied so that it overlaps the edges of the dressing underneath to an appreciable extent.

Washing of Wounds should not be done, but iodine solution should be applied by using sterilised swabs. These should be used once only and thrown away.

Burns.—The immediate application of a dressing is important in the case of a burn, as the immediate exclusion of air alleviates pain. The sterilised wool in the box can be used for this purpose, but special burn dressings consisting of lint impregnated with picric acid, are included in the outfit in cases where burns are likely to occur. The use of oil and grease should be avoided. When the burn is caused by a strong acid or caustic, the burn should be thoroughly flooded with water before using the sterilised dressing.

Injuries to the Eye.—Two kinds of injury have to be provided for.

(a) The presence of a foreign body.

The only First Aid permissible for this is to brush the eye gently with a brush carrying a little of the No. 1 solution mentioned in the First Aid leaflet, so that pain is relieved and the foreign body if possible brushed from the eye. Any further treatment must be given by a doctor, and no attempt should be made to remove the foreign body by any other means.

(b) A burn caused by splashes of acids or caustics.

In this case the eye must be thoroughly washed out with sterilised water, after which some drops of No. 2 solution mentioned in the First Aid leaflet should be dropped into it.

No injury to the eye should be neglected, whether it appears serious or not.

AMBULANCE ROOM.

The provision of an Ambulance Room is required under the Orders where 500 or more persons are employed. The accommodation, site, general construction, equipment and the provision for transport to hospital will depend upon the number of persons it is required to serve.

The Ambulance Room must be a separate room used only for the purpose of treatment and rest, with a floor space of not less than 100 square feet, smooth, hard and impervious walls and floor, and with ample means of natural and artificial lighting. It must contain at least—a glazed sink with hot and cold water always available ; a table with a smooth top ; means for sterilising instruments ; a supply of suitable dressings, bandages and splints ; a couch, and a stretcher.

A very complete illustrated brochure on the whole subject, from which the above abridged extracts have been taken, should be obtained by all to whom Section 7 (1) of the Police, Factories, &c. (Miscellaneous Provisions) Act applies. It can be obtained from His Majesty's Stationery Office or from St. John Ambulance Association, price 9d. net; by post, 10½d.

INDEX

K